Psychotherapy in India
Past, Present and Future

Psychotherapy in India
Past, Present and Future

Indian Psychiatric Society Publication

Editors

Geetha Desai MBBS MD PhD
Professor
Department of Psychiatry
National Institute of Mental Health and Neurosciences (NIMHANS)
Bengaluru, Karnataka, India

Vinay Kumar MD
Consultant Psychiatrist
Manoved Mind Hospital and Research Centre
Patna, Bihar, India
President, Indian Psychiatric Society

Pratap Sharan
MBBS MD (Psychiatry) PhD
Professor
Department of Psychiatry
All India Institute of Medical Sciences
New Delhi, India
Chairperson, Indian Psychiatric Society
Psychotherapy Specialty Section

Salman Akhtar
MBBS MD (Psychiatry) ABPN (USA) DLFAPA (USA)
Emeritus Professor
Department of Psychiatry
Jefferson Medical College
Philadelphia, PA, USA

JAYPEE BROTHERS MEDICAL PUBLISHERS
The Health Sciences Publisher
New Delhi | London

Jaypee Brothers Medical Publishers (P) Ltd

Headquarters

Jaypee Brothers Medical Publishers (P) Ltd
EMCA House, 23/23-B
Ansari Road, Daryaganj
New Delhi 110 002, India
Landline: +91-11-23272143, +91-11-23272703
+91-11-23282021, +91-11-23245672
Email: jaypee@jaypeebrothers.com

Corporate Office

Jaypee Brothers Medical Publishers (P) Ltd
4838/24, Ansari Road, Daryaganj
New Delhi 110 002, India
Phone: +91-11-43574357
Fax: +91-11-43574314
Email: jaypee@jaypeebrothers.com

Overseas Office

JP Medical Ltd
83 Victoria Street, London
SW1H 0HW (UK)
Phone: +44 20 3170 8910
Fax: +44 (0)20 3008 6180
Email: info@jpmedpub.com

Website: www.jaypeebrothers.com
Website: www.jaypeedigital.com

Inquiries for bulk sales may be solicited at: jaypee@jaypeebrothers.com

Psychotherapy in India: Past, Present and Future

First Edition: **2024**

ISBN: 978-93-5696-739-7

Printed in India

Contributors

Advait Dixit MD (Psychiatry)
Senior Resident
Department of Psychiatry
National Institute of Mental Health and Neurosciences (NIMHANS)
Bengaluru, Karnataka, India

Alok Sarin MBBS MD
Senior Consultant
Department of Psychiatry
Sitaram Bhartia Institute of Science and Research
New Delhi, India

Ananya Mahapatra MBBS MD DNB
Specialist
Department of Psychiatry
Dr Baba Saheb Ambedkar Hospital and Medical College
New Delhi, India

Arundhati Gairola MD
Senior Resident
Department of Psychiatry
King George's Medical University
Lucknow, Uttar Pradesh, India

Basant Pradhan MD
Professor
Department of Psychiatry and Pediatrics
Cooper Medical School of Rowan University
Camden, NJ, USA

Chhitij Srivastava
MD DNB MRCPsych CCT
Consultant Child and Adolescent Psychiatrist
Allahabad Child Development Centre
Prayagraj, Uttar Pradesh, India
Research Affiliate at Institute of Psychiatry, King's College London
London, UK

Gagan Hans MD (Psychiatry)
Additional Professor
Department of Psychiatry
All India Institute of Medical Sciences
New Delhi, India

Geetha Desai MBBS MD PhD
Professor
Department of Psychiatry
National Institute of Mental Health and Neurosciences (NIMHANS)
Bengaluru, Karnataka, India

Krishna Prasad Muliyala
MD (Psychiatry)
Professor
Department of Psychiatry
National Institute of Mental Health and Neurosciences (NIMHANS)
Bengaluru, Karnataka, India

Muralidharan Kesavan MD
Professor
Department of Psychiatry
National Institute of Mental Health and Neurosciences (NIMHANS)
Bengaluru, Karnataka, India

Neil Altman PhD
Faculty of Psychology
William Alanson White Institute
Cambridge, MA, USA

Nitesh Painuly
MBBS MD PG Diploma in Psychodynamic Psychotherapy Diploma in Groupwork Practice MBACP (Accrd.)
Consultant Psychiatrist
Department of Medical Psychotherapy
Personality Disorder Service and Community Eating Disorder Service
Devon Partnership NHS Trust
Exeter, UK

Pavithra Jayasankar MBBS MD (Psychiatry) PDF (Neuropsychiatry)
Assistant Professor
Department of Psychiatry
National Institute of Mental Health and Neurosciences (NIMHANS)
Bengaluru, Karnataka, India

Pratap Sharan
MBBS MD (Psychiatry) PhD
Professor
Department of Psychiatry
All India Institute of Medical Sciences
New Delhi, India
Chairperson, Indian Psychiatric Society Psychotherapy Specialty Section

Salman Akhtar
MBBS MD (Psychiatry) ABPN (USA) DLFAPA (USA)
Emeritus Professor
Department of Psychiatry
Jefferson Medical College
Philadelphia, PA, USA

Sanjeev Jain MBBS DPM MD
Emeritus Professor
Department of Psychiatry
National Institute of Mental Health and Neurosciences (NIMHANS)
Bengaluru, Karnataka, India

Satish Reddy MD
Diplomate, American Board of Psychiatry
Diplomate, American Board of Internal Medicine
American Board of Internal Medicine
Faculty, Columbia University Psychoanalytic Center
New York, NY

Satish Suhas MD
Assistant Professor
Department of Psychiatry
National Institute of Mental Health and Neurosciences (NIMHANS)
Bengaluru, Karnataka, India

Sumegha Mittal MD (Psychiatry)
Senior Resident
Department of Psychiatry
All India Institute of Medical Sciences
New Delhi, India

Vinay Kumar MD
Consultant Psychiatrist
Manoved Mind Hospital and Research Centre
Patna, Bihar, India
President, Indian Psychiatric Society

Vivek Agarwal MD
Professor and Head
Department of Psychiatry
King George's Medical University
Lucknow, Uttar Pradesh, India

Indian Psychiatric Society

If we go by public perception, all psychiatrists are basically psychotherapists, but when we look toward our competencies, we realize that only a few psychiatrists are true psychotherapists and most of us have some amount of theoretical knowledge only. This is basically due to two reasons. The first and most important is extensive research in biological psychiatry leading to psychopharmacological revolution, and the second is lack of training in psychotherapy due to a severe scarcity of trainers. Many psychiatrists have the notion that psychotherapy demands too much time and clients may find it cumbersome and expensive therapy. But those who have got training opportunities or have an orientation toward and insight in psychology realize that psychotherapeutic understanding makes you not only better psychiatrists but also better human beings by kindling not so active empathy and compassion.

The Indian Psychiatric Society has always realized the importance of this discipline and has tried organizing training workshops by experts from India and abroad. The idea of "Psychotherapy in India: Past, Present and Future" also took birth and shape during similar workshops by Professor Salman Akhtar. This book is an attempt to understand the past, present, and future of psychotherapy in India, and has substantial scientific information and evidence to enrich and inspire the readers.

The Indian Psychiatric Society is thankful to all the editors and contributors for devoting time and hard work. We are indebted to Professor Salman Akhtar who always accepts our invitation for conducting psychotherapy workshop and has helped Indian Psychiatric Society (IPS) in bringing out this book with his intellectual inputs and master editorial skills.

We congratulate the Publication Committee led by Professor Anil Kakunje for another milestone book. The credit for the beautiful cover goes to Padma Shree Shyam Sharma who gave us permission to use his unique artwork. We express our gratitude to him. We are thankful to Shri Jitendar P Vij (Group Chairman), Mr Ankit Vij (Managing Director), Ms Chetna Malhotra

(Senior Director—Professional Publishing, Marketing, and Business Development), Ms Pragati Singh (Development Editor), and the entire team of M/s Jaypee Brothers Medical Publishers (P) Ltd, New Delhi, India, for their efforts.

Vinay Kumar	**Laxmikant Rathi**	**Arabinda Brahma**
President	Vice President	Hon. General Secretary

Message from the Publication Committee

Indian Psychiatric Society

It is a matter of great pleasure to write a message for the book *Psychotherapy in India: Past, Present and Future,* a growing field.

It is heartening to see Indian Psychiatric Society (IPS) coming up with a lot of books on Psychiatry; it is not just textbooks but books on many specialty topics and niche areas. There is a need to get an in-depth knowledge of each illness population, treatment modalities with special emphasis on the Indian context; not just for students but also for all mental health professionals and researchers.

Psychiatry is now not limited to treating mainly severe mental illness in mental hospitals. Psychiatrists now handle varied illnesses, and many are related to children, adolescents, women, perinatal period, geriatric population and so on. There are a large number of people who are seen as out-patients and request psychotherapy. I feel glad to highlight that this unique book *Psychotherapy in India: Past, Present and Future* covers every aspect in great detail by experts in the field.

The lead editor who is my teacher too; Professor Dr Geetha Desai and her team have put in real hard work to make this book a reality. The Publication Committee congratulates them on bringing out this book which is the need of the hour.

I on behalf of the Publication Committee thank the IPS Office Bearers for their continued support and co-operation. I also thank Shri Jitendar P Vij (Group Chairman), Mr Ankit Vij (Managing Director), Ms Chetna Malhotra (Senior Director—Professional Publishing, Marketing, and Business Development), Ms Pragati Singh (Development Editor), and the entire team of M/s Jaypee Brothers Medical Publishers (P) Ltd, New Delhi, India, for their efforts. I am sure this book will be a hugely popular and will make a mark in the field of Psychotherapy.

Long Live IPS!

Anil Kakunje
Chairperson

Sai Krishna Tikka
Co-Chairperson

Snehil Gupta
Convener

Shahul Ameen
EC Representative

Mrugesh Vaishnav
Advisor

Preface

Psychotherapy has been considered a treatment modality for mental health conditions as a stand-alone treatment as well as an adjunct to other treatments. Over the years, many schools of psychotherapy have been proposed, tested, and used for treatment. There has been a vast difference in psychotherapy practice across various regions of the world.

Talking specifically of India, one is struck by the hugely contradictory situation of great need for psychotherapy on the one hand and relative paucity of organized education of psychiatric trainees in this realm. The former is acutely felt in large metropolitan areas of the country (e.g., Mumbai, New Delhi, Kolkata, Chennai, Bengaluru, Hyderabad) and reflects the unmistakable decline of joint and extended families, change in patterns of child-rearing, increased aloneness in childhood, and the overall fraying of interpersonal warmth and connectedness in busy and increasingly market-oriented societies. The latter is discernible via the meagerness of formal didactics in psychotherapy, the excessive 'medicalization' of psychiatry, and the absence of formal and informal links between psychiatrists and non-medical psychotherapists and psychoanalysts. Surely, something needs to be done.

This book *Psychotherapy in India: Past, Present and Future* was planned to compile the psychotherapy work in India. The book begins with an exploration of the history of psychotherapy in India. The book has two sections, and section 1 "Inquiring Voices from the Region", delves into the training of psychotherapy in India, challenges of psychotherapy with different populations and addressing psychotherapy in India globally. Section 2 "Helpful Echoes from the Indian Diaspora" highlighting the cultural and spiritual components in psychotherapy. Section 2 also highlights the journey of therapists who trained in India and how India has surfaced in their psychotherapy practice. The concluding part of the book pens down the future direction of psychotherapy in India. This book is neither a textbook on psychotherapy, nor does it address the different schools of therapy. This book is being written with the hope that it generates interest in psychotherapy practice in India. More importantly, its aim is to mobilize academic dialogue, empirical research, evaluation and development of fresh training approaches, and, hopefully, an interdisciplinary orientation to considering the future of psychotherapy in India.

Geetha Desai
Pratap Sharan
Vinay Kumar
Salman Akhtar

Contents

Epilogue

Prologue

1 CHAPTER History of Psychotherapy in India

Pratap Sharan, Ananya Mahapatra, Alok Sarin, Sanjeev Jain

ABSTRACT

This chapter delves into the history of psychotherapy in India, tracing its origins to ancient Indian traditions and integrating Western psychological concepts. It explores psychotherapy's development from the Vedic period to its formalization during the British colonial era and examines its contemporary applications in modern mental health care. The chapter examines key figures and cultural adaptations in Indian psychotherapy; the advent of therapies like behavior therapy and cognitive behavioral therapy; and provides a critical analysis of the development of psychotherapy in India. It finally emphasizes the need for addressing social issues like poverty and disparity in the Indian psychotherapy framework.

Keywords: History, Psychotherapy, Universalism vs. Exceptionalism, Critical analysis

INTRODUCTION

The history of psychotherapy in India reflects centuries of cultural, philosophical, and epistemological evolution. Taking root in the ancient traditional systems of the Indian subcontinent, what is called psychotherapy in India has undergone a remarkable transformation that has resulted in the assimilation of Western psychological theories and concepts derived from Eastern philosophy (related to the interconnectedness of mind, body, and spirit) and indigenous practices.

The introduction of Western psychotherapy schools in India occurred during the British colonial period within an overarching imposition of Western healthcare systems, educational institutions, and socio-cultural practices within traditional Indian society. It set the stage for laying the foundations of present psychotherapeutic methods in India.

This chapter aims to describe the evolution of psychotherapy in India from its origins in Vedic and Ayurvedic traditions, traversing through the influence of Western psychological paradigms brought to India during the colonial era, leading to the establishment of formalized psychotherapeutic practices, and its contemporary manifestations in the context of modern mental health care.

ANCIENT PERIOD

Frank JD (1973) gave a broad definition of psychotherapy as a "type of social influence exerted by a trained and socially sanctioned healer on a person or persons who suffer and are seeking relief, through a series of defined contacts." From this vantage point, the principles of psychotherapy can be discerned in the age-old practices and texts of traditional societies.[1] The Bhagavad Gita is often quoted as one of the earliest documented texts incorporating core psychotherapy principles as we understand it today.[2] Krishna's dialogue with Arjuna on the battlefield of Kurukshetra contains insights into the human psyche and pathways to mental peace and self-realization. Aimed at resolving Arjuna's "internal conflict," the dialogue employs strategies comparable to contemporary psychotherapy practices such as cognitive behavior therapy, grief therapy, motivation enhancement, and interpersonal and supportive psychotherapies.[3]

The Atharvaveda, in its descriptions of the management of mental ailments, describes a nonpharmacological treatment modality called "Sattvavajaya Chikitsa," which has been considered the equivalent of psychotherapy in Ayurveda.[4] Sattvavajaya Chikitsa, devised by Acharya Charaka, who is revered as the pioneer of Ayurvedic medicine, employs a psychospiritual strategy that is designed to steer the mind (Manas) away from harmful distractions (Ahita Artha), such as undesirable thoughts and perceptions.[5] Its techniques focus on the affected individuals' intelligence, consciousness, memory, and spiritual aspects; and aim to stimulate consciousness, and alter the maladaptive thoughts/actions, in ways like modern psychotherapeutic practices.[6] Similarly, while elaborating on the Buddha's discourses, Dr JS Neki demonstrated that even though they do not study the mind as a clinical entity, many of Buddha's dialogues specifically aim to bring about changes in consciousness and our awareness of our feelings; and modify one's relations with one's natural and social surroundings. Dr Neki commented that "one cannot but designate them as 'psychotherapies' in a wider sense."[7] Similarly, the Guru Granth Sahib, which is the primary religious text for Sikhs, describes emotions in everyday life, such as happiness, sadness, anger, and hatred; as well as more serious mental health issues, such as depression; and prescribes certain spiritual and therapeutic ways to relieve problems of emotional nature.[8] Dr Vidya Sagar regularly prescribed recitation of some specified portions of religious scriptures like the Gita and Sukhmani Sahib to his Hindu and Sikh clients respectively, as an aid to psychotherapy.[9]

India has several alternative systems of medicine, which contemplate types of living that would promote health including psychological health. Ayurveda conceives a set of emotions like Kama (Lust), Krodha (Anger), Lobha (Greed), Moha (Affection), Irsya (Jealousy), Harsa (Happiness), Visada (Grief), Cittodveqa (Anxiety), etc., as basic components of psychopathology and suggests treatments like replacing the pathogenic emotions with the opposite ones.[4] The technique of replacement of emotion is compared to shuttling in Gestalt therapy. Similarly, the Siddha system of medicine practiced in Southern India has a 'treatment method' called 'Mantiram' that lays emphasis on treating the 'psyche' by removing unhealthy thoughts, behavior and postures, and replacing them with good thoughts (*emayam*), traits (*niyamam*), and postures (*asanam*).[10] Islamic medicine also stressed the need for the understanding of human mental health. Medieval Muslim psychotherapy provided moral treatment, music therapy and occupational therapy among other methods.[11] Muslim influence led to the development of the Unani system of medicine in India.[12]

COLONIAL PERIOD

The introduction of the Western psychological school of thought as a scientific discipline within India occurred for the first time in the 19th century during British rule, within a larger context of structured integration of Western educational systems, scientific thinking, and cultural exchange across the Indian urban society.[13] The establishment of universities in major cities such as Calcutta (Kolkata), Bombay (Mumbai), and Madras (Chennai) during the mid to late 19th century was pivotal in this regard since these universities began to include Western curricula, which included the study of philosophy and, later, psychology. The official introduction of Western psychology to India is often credited to the setting up the Department of Philosophy with a focus on psychology at Calcutta University in the early 20th century.[14] This was followed by the introduction of experimental psychology at Calcutta University in 1916 by Narendra Nath Sengupta, a student of Hugo Münsterberg, a pioneer in applied psychology, upon his return from Harvard University.[15]

Between the First World War and Independence in 1947 Indian personnel started being placed at senior levels in the Indian Medical Service. A notable example of Indian leadership in mental healthcare services during this period was JE Dhunjibhoy at the Ranchi Indian Mental Hospital. One of the forms of treatment in which Dhunjibhoy showed a degree of interest was psychoanalysis.[16] Between 1920s and 1940s there were two trends concerning the relationship between psychoanalysis and the colonial setting. Owen Berkeley-Hill (1897–1944), a British medical officer and psychoanalyst, was emblematic of the first trend that was essentially Freudian. Girindrasekhar Bose represented the second more hybrid trend[17] that integrated Western psychoanalytical methodologies and theories with Indian philosophical ideas.

Girindrasekhar Bose founded the Indian Psychoanalytic Society in 1922. After Bose earned an MBBS degree from Calcutta Medical College in 1910, he studied psychology in the newly opened Department of Psychology at Calcutta University. He obtained a master's degree in psychology in 1917.[18] Credited with formally introducing Sigmund Freud's analytically-oriented psychotherapy in India and starting a training program in psychoanalysis at Calcutta University in 1930, Bose was known to be in regular correspondence with Freud. In 1921, Bose began his correspondence with Freud and sent him his book *The Concept of Repression,* which received a favorable comment from Freud: *"It was a great and pleasant surprise that the first book on a psychoanalytic subject which comes to us from...India displays so good knowledge of psychoanalysis, so deep an insight into its difficulties and so much of deep-going original thought".*[19]

Bose also attempted to synthesize Freudian psychoanalytic principles with thoughts from Indian scriptures and traditional Indian knowledge systems, as documented in his publications, such as Purana Prabesh (Introduction to Purana Shastras).[20] In 1940, he established the Lumbini Park Mental Hospital, which was a private hospital and clinic managed by the Indian Psychoanalytical Society, where psychoanalytical therapy was emphasized as one of the forms of treatment in its initial years till it attained mental hospital status under the Lunacy Act in 1952.[21]

Dr D Satyanand, who trained under O Berkley Hill in 1934, attempted to synthesize psychoanalytical principles and dream analysis with Indian mysticism and religious symbolism. He analyzed dreams from the psychoanalytic (Freudian, Adlerian, and Jungian perspectives) and 'oriental reminiscence state' (e.g., mystic, "samadhi", and religious) perspectives.[22] In his analysis, which he named "soul analysis," Satyanand emphasized the dreamer's cultural context, suggesting that dreams' meanings are deeply rooted in one's cultural background and personal experiences, thereby enriching the global understanding of dream analysis and reflecting an amalgamation of Western psychoanalytic theories and Indian philosophical perspectives.

Post-World War II, a few qualified psychotherapists practiced different forms of psychotherapy in the country. For example, Dr Vasavada from Jodhpur practiced Jungian psychotherapy; Dr Satyanand from Ranchi, and later Delhi, was a Kleinian, and Dr Hoch, who worked at Lucknow, was described as an existentialist.[23] However, psychotherapeutic methods failed to become firmly rooted in India as a standard method of treatment.

POST-COLONIAL PERIOD

Development of psychotherapy (and psychiatry) around independence was linked to transnational networks and philanthropy. Two psychiatric institutions were established in the 1950s, the Nur Manzil Psychiatric Center in Lucknow (by E Stanley Hall), and the Mental Health Centre at the Christian Medical College, Vellore, Tamil Nadu. These were led by among others, Erna Hoch (Swiss Psychiatrist) and Margaret Foyle (British Psychoanalyst) at Nur Manzil; and Florence Nichols (Canadian Psychiatrist and

Psychoanalyst) and Rose Chacko (Child Psychiatrist) at the Christian Medical College. Both institutions aimed to provide low-cost treatment to Indian communities, and both were involved in the advancement of new family and drug therapies.[12,24]

The history of psychoanalysis in the postcolonial period of India is centered in Ahmedabad, with influential figures such as Erik Erikson and Sudhir Kakar playing pivotal roles. Smt Kamalini Sarabhai, who underwent psychoanalytic training at the British Psychoanalytical Society (BPAS) and the Tavistock Clinic, London, developed the BM Institute in Ahmedabad, where Erik Erikson is said to have extensively researched Mahatma Gandhi's role in the 1918 Ahmedabad strike and his methods of social reform, by conducting interviews with Gandhi's close associates and studying his writings. This research culminated in Erikson's psychobiography titled 'Gandhi's Truth,' which delves into Gandhi's psychological and philosophical beliefs.[25]

In the late 1960s, Erik Erikson is said to have identified the potential in Sudhir Kakar during his visit to India. This encounter led Kakar to pursue training in Freudian-Eriksonian analysis in Germany. After his training, Kakar returned to India and developed a unique psychoanalytic approach that was deeply intertwined with India's cultural and spiritual fabric.[26]

Kakar's work is characterized by its emphasis on the relationship between culture and the unconscious. He observed that while Western psychoanalysis is often focused on the individual, Indian psychology is influenced by a myriad of factors, including class, culture, and specifically Hindu traditions. His approach sought to blend psychoanalytic principles with Hindu religious mythology and mysticism, aiming to Indianize psychoanalysis culturally.[27]

Recently, Santanu Biswas, a Literature Professor at Jadavpur University, introduced Lacanian psychoanalysis to India in Kolkata around 2012.[26] His approach to psychoanalysis was marked by a critique of political discourses of power and dominant ideology, using psychoanalysis as an antidogmatic tool. He addresses complex social issues such as caste, gender, and religious identities and their psychic effects like shame and guilt.[28]

Discontent with Western Psychotherapy

Despite the initial interest garnered for Western analytical schools of psychotherapy in the post-independence era, Neki observed that "*the practice of modern psychotherapy in India has by no means been the analytic kind; it has mostly been an 'incidental,' 'common-sense,' 'supportive,' and 'superficial' kind, not conforming consistently to any particular school, but subserving expediency in the treatment of psychiatric patients and employed mostly as an adjunct to somatotherapy.*"[7] A survey conducted in 1973 by Varma and Ghosh on the practice of psychotherapy among the Fellows of the Indian Psychiatric

Society reported that only 17% of them were using any psychological method of treatment.[29]

The failure of psychotherapy to take root in India was largely laid on its foreignness. It was emphasized that Western psychotherapy does not work well in the Indian context due to the significant cultural and social gap between therapists and their clients, which leads to communication barriers and a lack of shared understanding.[30] It is believed that applying Western psychotherapeutic models that are primarily focused on the individual (intrapsychic dynamic models and ego structure) is challenging within the framework of a collectivistic society.

Since the 1960s, discontent with Western models of psychotherapy and the limitations of their applicability to the Indian population has been more vocally expressed. Varma reported that the Indian population possessed seven distinct features that limited the relevance of the Western type of psychotherapy.[31] These include: (1) Dependence/interdependence, (2) lack of psychological sophistication, (3) social distance between the doctor and the patient, (4) religious belief in rebirth and fatalism, (5) guilt attributed to misdeeds in past life, (6) confidentiality, and (7) personal responsibility in decision-making. Amongst these, he cited dependence/interdependence (a marker of collectivism) in Indian patients on/with other family members as the foremost of the seven difficulties in carrying out dynamic and individual-oriented psychotherapy. Surya and Jayaram have also pointed out that Indian patients are more dependent than their Western counterparts, which makes it difficult for therapists to apply the orthodox Western models of psychotherapy to their patients.[32] *"As compared to his Western counterpart, the Indian patient is more ready to expect and accept dependency relationships; more ready to accept overt situational support, less ready to seek intrapsychic explanations; more insistent and importunate about personal needs and time; more ready to disregard ego-bounds and involve the therapist in direct role relationship; and finally, his ideal or idealized support is the good joint-family."*

Neki, in his analysis of the ideas of confidentiality and privacy within the Indian context, expressed the view that these concepts are virtually nonexistent in Indian socio-cultural norms and further went on to suggest that the notion of privacy could lead to isolation in a society where interdependence is highly valued.[33]

Attempts to Formulate Indian Forms of Psychotherapy

There have been efforts to incorporate traditional Indian philosophy into psychotherapeutic practices. Surya and Jayaram noted that Indian mythological tales could be utilized as psychotherapeutic tools since the Indian client would more readily allude to traditional references for orientation and identification; for example, the legend of Savitri could serve as a psychotherapeutic model.[32] Verma conceptualized psychotherapy as an 'interpersonal method for alleviating suffering,' tracing its origins to Buddha's teachings and highlighting the relevance of Karma and Dharma in therapy.[34] Satyanand used the Shaivite symbolic models in an indigenous adaptation of analytical psychotherapy.[35] Neki explored the use of various Indian concepts, including nirvana, and discussed the Guru-Chela relationship as an indigenous therapeutic model for psychotherapy.

Carstairs G (1965) was the first to suggest that a model of psychotherapy built on the framework of the traditional Guru-Chela concept might be tenable for the Indian population.[36] In his landmark paper published in 1973, Neki elaborated upon the idea of the Guru-Chela relationship as a novel psychotherapeutic paradigm.[37] In this paradigm, the therapist (Guru) is regarded and respected as a knowledgeable mentor who imparts wisdom and guidance. The paradigm shifts away from the more detached, clinical approach typical of Western psychotherapy, and envisages a more personalized and empathetic bond between the therapist and the patient.

More recently, Wig introduced the 'Hanuman complex' as a way of aiding both patients and doctors in understanding the psychotherapy process.[38] Quoting the increasing use of stories, metaphors, allegories, and narrative practices in psychotherapies across different cultures, especially in European countries such as Norway, Finland, etc., Wig suggested that we can use our rich mythological stories and symbols and explore their applicability in therapy. He exemplified the same through the "Hanuman Complex," as a culturally contextualized way to understand and address issues related to self-esteem and self-perception.

These efforts at integrating Indian traditional concepts with modern psychotherapeutic techniques and devising novel psychotherapeutic paradigms suited for the Indian population, did not succeeded in taking root in the mainstream practice of psychotherapy. This may be because these psychotherapeutic practices are steeped in traditional, philosophical, and religious concepts, which can sometimes be esoteric and challenging to comprehend for the elitist professionals and the common clients who do not belong to the 'high-culture'.[23] Ultimately, the validity of these concepts was not tested and alternative 'Indian psychotherapeutic framework(s)' did not get organized.[23,37]

By the late 1970s, psychoanalytically-oriented psychotherapy and its Indian adaptations began falling out of favor, and emerging therapies based on the principles of behaviorism, cognitive theory, social learning, etc., made their appearance in the Indian psychotherapy space.

Cognitive Behavioral Approaches

Behavior Therapy

Satyanand introduced behavior therapy, which was not a well-known form of psychological treatment during the sixties, to the Indian professional audience.[39] Behavior therapy as a newly emerging psychotherapeutic modality was initially critiqued by psychoanalytically-oriented therapists for targeting behavior modification without attempting to resolve the deep-seated intrapsychic conflict.[40] However, behavioral therapy stood out as the first psychological treatment approach that demonstrated its effectiveness through stringent scientific evaluation methods, such as randomized, placebo-controlled, double-blind studies. However, since its introduction as a psychotherapeutic technique in the 1970s till early 2010s, its use has mainly been eclectic, and without adequate focus on methodological rigor.[40]

Dr LP Varma established India's first behavior therapy unit in 1971 at the Central Institute of Psychiatry in Ranchi.[41] In addition to direct therapeutic services, the unit at the Central Institute of Psychiatry also played a crucial role in training and educating mental health professionals in behavior therapy techniques across India.

A review of papers published till 2009 revealed a noticeable overreliance on aversion techniques across a broad range of disorders, including hysteria, homosexuality, tremors, and titubation during the initial years.[40] Jacobson's Progressive Muscle Relaxation (JPMR) was so widely employed as a behavioral method, that it became synonymous with behavior therapy in India.[42]

Cognitive Behavior and Third Wave Therapies

Cognitive behavioral therapy (CBT) was introduced in India during the 1970s as a part of a broader movement towards incorporating contemporary psychotherapeutic techniques into mental health practice.[40] The introduction coincided with an increased global exchange of knowledge and the establishment of more formal training and education in psychology within the country. In the last two decades, CBT has been increasingly utilized as a primary psychotherapeutic method for the psychological treatment of various mental disorders in India. There is an emerging trend in corporate sectors to hire industrial/organizational psychologists skilled in CBT to address work-life balance issues among employees.[43]

As with psychoanalytical psychotherapy, there were some doubts regarding the applicability of 'western' cognitive therapy in the Indian setting, and the need for an indigenous adaptation was emphasized.[44] However, with deepening globalization, the emphasis on cultural exclusivity in the psychotherapeutic discourse has gradually diminished.

The introduction of third-wave psychotherapies in India has marked a significant evolution in the field of psychotherapy in the last couple of decades. These therapies, which include Acceptance and Commitment Therapy (ACT), Dialectical Behavior Therapy (DBT), and Mindfulness-Based Cognitive Therapy (MBCT), focus on concepts like mindfulness, acceptance, and the understanding of one's thoughts and feelings in a nonjudgmental way. This shift reflects a broader, more holistic approach to mental health, emphasizing the importance of context and the individual's relationship with his/her thoughts and emotions.

The Indian Association for Cognitive Behaviour Therapy (IACBT) was established in 2016. It serves as a platform for students, professionals, and the consumers of mental health services to access evidence-based practice, research, and supervised training in CBT in India and establishing a 'network' of trained CBT experts in India (https://www.iacbt.org/).

DEVELOPMENTS IN CLINICAL PSYCHOLOGY

The emergence of psychology as a discipline occurred within the psychodynamic context during the colonial period, when the Indian Psychoanalytical Institute introduced a training program in clinical psychology.

In 1945, the University of Calcutta introduced an applied and abnormal psychology certificate course, and in 1951, Banaras Hindu University started a 1-year program in clinical psychology.[45] It is important to note that this predates the development of psychiatry as a profession or discipline within the medical curriculum in India.

During the late seventies, the founder President of the Indian Association of Clinical Psychologists, the late NN Sen, initiated a program at the Kashi Vidyapeeth. This and the applied psychology courses at the Aligarh Muslim University, and clinical psychology programs at the Karnatak University, Dharwar and SNDT Women's University, Mumbai, existed for a few years. Although efforts were made to provide the trainees in these programs with some exposure to clinical material, adequate clinical supervision proved challenging. In the face of reduced facilities to impart clinical skills, most programs remained low profile and less popular with the students, and in time, most became extinct.

In 1954, the Indian government established the All India Institute of Mental Health in Bangalore, renamed in 1974 as the National Institute of Mental Health and Neurosciences (NIMHANS). This institute introduced a Diploma in Medical and Social Psychology in 1960, which later transitioned to a MPhil program in Medical and Social Psychology (1978) and still later into a MPhil program in Clinical Psychology. Similar training programs were launched at the Postgraduate Training Centre in Ranchi in 1962 and at the BM Institute in Ahmedabad in 1973.[46]

In this period (1955–1970), the emphasis shifted to diagnostic assessment particularly at the newly established All India Institute of Mental Health (AIIMH) and subsequent similar mental health establishments. Things did not change much despite the introduction of a Behavior Therapy Unit in CIP, Ranchi. A notable imbalance in the professional duties of clinical psychologists has been highlighted in such settings, where diagnostic tasks were overly prioritized at the expense of therapeutic, educational, and research responsibilities.[46]

With the establishment of Rehabilitation Council of India as a statutory body in 1993, clinical psychology became a state-recognized profession.

CRITIQUE OF THE HISTORICAL DEVELOPMENTS IN PSYCHOTHERAPY IN INDIA

Epistemological Critique

Colonization led to the hegemony of the Western "scientific" system and exclusion of 'Indian sciences' as serious epistemological contenders. During the early postcolonial period, Indian scholars felt like 'victims of epistemological violence'—the denigration and belittling of one's categories of knowledge and understanding. This understandably led to opposition to colonial systems of knowledge,[17,26] however, most efforts harked back rather than onward and ultimately proved futile.[23]

Chakraborty (2007) subtly debunks authors like Varma, Wig, and Neki's arguments on lack of psychological sophistication of 'Indian' subjects; and regrets the implied 'colonial' subservience in the guise of token 'anticolonialism.' She states, "*Colonialists and anthropologists (for a time) had been telling the world from the early days, (e.g., Freud's primal horde) that the Indian ego is not individual but group-ego, it remains merged with the group or community, and the individual self is 'bonded.' According to such viewpoints Indians usually cannot act independently, like children whose ego is 'infantile and immature.'*"[47] The *Guruvadi* inclination in Indian psychotherapy has been criticized for being predominantly hierarchical and top down and being reflective of both colonial and feudal traditions.[26]

The questions on feasibility of applying western psychotherapy in India has been criticized as being impossible to answer, as each of the concepts 'Western,' 'India,' and 'Psychotherapy' are heterogeneous.[23] Since psychotherapy ultimately focuses more on the singularity of the subject than their cultural genericity, Prabhu (1988) states that 'western' psychotherapies are not out of place in the Indian setup if therapists develop the sensitivities to cater to the individuality of the client.

The way forward may be to creatively assimilate, rather than 'overcome,' the opposition of, us and them, through significant epistemic border-crossing and interdisciplinary methodologies.[48] Some of the pioneering psychoanalysts of India like Girindrashekhar Bose and Sudhir Kakar attempted to culturally Indianize psychoanalysis.[26] And the third wave cognitive behavioral approaches are transversal in their approach.

Pragmatic Critique

Professionalization

The ethical code of professional bodies specifically direct that professionals should practice only within the area of their competence based on training and experience to protect patients, clients, students, research participants, and others from harm. The professionalization of psychotherapy in India began in the 20th century with the creation of the Indian Psychoanalytic Society and its supervised training program. The next significant development has been the formation of the Indian Association for Cognitive Behaviour Therapy (IACBT) in 2016. However, the Indian Psychoanalytic Society has not integrated itself with the mainstream mental health enterprise in India and does not seem to be gaining many adherents; while the IACBT does not offer a course that would train a full-fledged professional psychotherapist.

Training of Psychotherapists

Psychotherapy training involves different levels of proficiency. Practitioners can be trained to become psychotherapy supervisors, psychotherapists, psychotherapeutically informed mental health professionals, and psychotherapeutically informed other health/wellness professional/workers.

To practice as a psychotherapist in the West, one must undergo specialized training in psychotherapy, often for 2–6 or more years (depending on the requirements of various professional/statutory bodies) before one is accredited as a psychotherapist who can offer professional psychotherapy services. Psychotherapists must undergo further training as supervisors, before gaining accreditation/recognition as psychotherapy trainers. These levels of training are available only with the Indian Psychoanalytic Society in India.

Since psychotherapeutic intervention are widely needed, psychotherapy training should be mandatory in all courses for mental health professionals. At present such training is quite rudimentary in courses offered by most psychiatric training centers in India.[49] The Rehabilitation Council of India's Master of Philosophy (MPhil) Clinical Psychology curriculum includes an introduction to psychotherapy and practice with clinical supervision in psychotherapy for specified number of hours. Statutory bodies like the Medical Council of India and Nursing Council of India should mandate uniform psychotherapy training as essential course requirement for other mental health professionals like psychiatrists, and psychiatric nurses.

Beyond this there is also a need to develop (limited) psychotherapy training (and refresher) courses for health/wellness professionals and workers; and to develop self-help psychotherapeutic materials for the population.

SUMMARY/CONCLUSION

The history of psychotherapy in India encompasses a blend of ancient cultural practices and Western psychological theories. It traces its roots to classical texts like the Bhagavad Gita and traditional Indian systems like Ayurveda. The British colonial period marked the introduction of Western psychotherapy, leading to a synthesis of Eastern and Western approaches. However, the evolution of psychotherapy in India reveals a significant gap in addressing social issues. Unlike Western psychotherapy, which has dynamically evolved in response to societal challenges, Indian psychotherapy has been less responsive to deep-rooted problems like poverty, social disparities, communalism, gender, and caste. This indicates a need for Indian psychotherapy to develop a more socially aware and culturally sensitive approach, integrating the understanding of these complex social dynamics into therapeutic practices.

REFERENCES

1. Frank JD. Persuasion and Healing, 2nd edition. Baltimore, MD: Johns Hopkins University Press; 1973.
2. Balodhi JP, Keshavan MS. Bhagavad Gita and psychotherapy. Asian J Psychiatr. 2011;4(4):300-2.
3. Bhatia SC, Madabushi J, Kolli V, Bhatia SK, Madaan V. The Bhagavad Gita and contemporary psychotherapies. Indian J Psychiatr. 2013;55(Suppl 2):S315-21.
4. Behere PB, Das A, Yadav R, Behere AP. Ayurvedic concepts related to psychotherapy. Indian J Psychiatr. 2013;55(Suppl 2):S310-14.
5. Tripathi JS. Dimensions of Sattvavajaya Chikitsa (Ayurvedic psychotherapy) and their clinical applications. Ann Ayurvedic Med. 2012;1(1-2):31-8.
6. Bagali SS, Baragi UC, Deshmukh RA. Concept of Satwavajaya Chikitsa (Psychotherapy). J. Ayurveda Integr Med Sci. 2016;1(01):56-63.
7. Neki JS. Psychotherapy in India: past, present, and future. Am J Psychother. 1975;29(1):92-100.
8. Kalra G, Bhui K, Bhugra D. Does *Guru Granth Sahib* describe depression? Indian Psychiatr. 2013;55(Suppl 2):S195-200.
9. Singh K. In pursuit of happiness. Indian J Psychiatr. 1983;25(1):7-13.
10. Ottilingam S, Murthy T, Raghavan V. Mental health: concepts and treatment in the Siddha (Tamil) system of medicine. Asean J Psychiatr. 2015;16. [online] Available from https://www.aseanjournalofpsychiatry.org/articles/mental-health-concepts-and-treatment-in-the-siddha-tamil-system-of-medicine.pdf. [Last accessed December, 2023]
11. Majeed A, Jameer KP. The contribution of Muslims and Islamic concepts: Rethinking and establishing the actual origin of concepts and thought in psychology. Int J Indian Psychol. 2017;4(2):96.

12. Jain S, Sarin A, van Ginneken N, Murthy P, Harding C, Chatrejee S. Psychiatry in India: Historical roots, development as a discipline and contemporary context. In. Minas H, Lewis M (Eds). Mental Health in Asia and the Pacific, International and Cultural Psychology. New York, Springer Science+Business Media; 2017. pp. 39-57.
13. Kakar S. Stories from Indian psychoanalysis: Context and text. In: Stighler JW, Shweder RA, Herdt G (Eds). Cultural Psychology: Essays on Comparative Human Development. New York: Cambridge University Press; 1990. pp. 427-45.
14. Sanyal N. History of Psychology at Calcutta University Across the Century. In: Misra G, Sanyal N, De S (Eds). Psychology in Modern India: Historical, Methodological, and Future Perspectives, Singapore, Springer Verlag; 2021. pp. 35-60.
15. Dalal AK. A journey back to the roots: Psychology in India. In: Cornelisson M, Misra G, Verma S (Eds). Foundations and Applications of Indian Psychology. New Delhi, Pearson; 2014. pp. 18-39.
16. Ernst W. Colonialism and transnational psychiatry: The development of an Indian mental hospital in British India (1925–1940). London: Anthem; 2013.
17. Boni, L. Interview with Ashis Nandy: psychoanalytic sociology and post-colonial predicament. In: Nandy A (Ed). Breakfast with Evil and Other Risky Ventures. The Non-Essential Ashis Nandy. New Delhi, Oxford University Press; 2021. pp. 229-48.
18. Misra G, Kumar M. Psychology in India: Retrospect and prospect. In: Misra G (Ed). Psychology in India (Theoretical and methodological developments), Vol. 4. New Delhi, Pearson; 2011. pp. 339-76.
19. Hartnack C. Vishnu on Freud's desk: Psychoanalysis in colonial India. Social Research: An International Quarterly. 1990;57:921-50.
20. Bose G. A new technique of psychoanalysis. Int J Psychoanal. 1931;12:387-8.
21. Hartnack C. Psychoanalysis in Bengal. In: Haetnack C (Ed). Psychoanalysis in Colonial India. New Delhi, Oxford University Press; 2001. pp. 87-119.
22. Jain S, Murthy P, Sarin A. The story of Satyanand. Indian J Psychiatry. 2015; 57(4):419.
23. Prabhu GG. Psychotherapy in India. Indian J Psychol Med. 1988;11(2):155-9.
24. Harding CG. The emergence of 'Christian psychiatry' in post-Independence India. Edinburgh Papers in South Asian Studies (Vol. 24). Edinburgh: Edinburgh University Centre for South Asian Studies; 2011.
25. Mehta R, Shah A, Vankar GK, Chauhan A, Bakre R. Golden roots to golden fruits of mental health in Gujarat. Indian J Psychiatr. 2018;60(Suppl 2):S227-235.
26. Rousselle D. Psychoanalysis in India? Duane Rousselle Interviews Arka Chattopadhyay. Eur J Psychoanal. 2022;9:2. [online] Available from http://bminstituteofmentalhealth.com/history/ [Last accessed December, 2023].
27. Kakar S. Psychoanalysis and Eastern spiritual healing traditions. J Anal Psychol. 2003;48(5):659-78.
28. Mishra AK. Shall the Twain Ever Meet? The cultural politics of psychoanalysis in India. In: Misra, G, Sanyal N, De S (Eds). Psychology in Modern India: Historical, Methodological, and Future Perspectives, Singapore, Springer Verlag; 2021. pp. 93-118.
29. Varma VK, Ghosh A. Psychotherapy as practiced by the Indian Psychiatrists. Indian J Psychiatr. 1976;18:177-86.
30. Shamasundar C. What kind of psychotherapy in the Indian setting? Indian J Psychiatr. 1979;21(1):34-8.

31. Manickam LS. Psychotherapy in India. Indian J Psychiatr. 2010;52(Suppl 1):S366-70.
32. Surya N, Jayaram S. Some basic considerations in the practice of psychotherapy in the Indian setting. Indian J Psychiatr. 1996;38(1):10-2.
33. Neki JS. Confidentiality, secrecy, and privacy in psychotherapy: Sociodynamic considerations. Indian J Psychiatr. 1992;34(3):171-3.
34. Varma VK. Present state of psychotherapy in India. Indian J Psychiatr. 1982;24(3):209-26.
35. Nand DS. A comparative study of scientific and religious psychotherapy with a special study of the role of the commonest shivite symbolic model in total psychoanalysis. Indian J Psychiatr. 1961;3(4):261-73.
36. Carstairs GM. Cultural elements in response to treatment. In: DeReack A, Porter P (Eds). Ciba Foundation Symposium on Trans-cultural Psychiatry. JA Churchill, London; 1965.
37. Neki JS. Gurū-Chelā relationship: The possibility of a therapeutic paradigm. Am J Orthopsychiatry. 1973;43(5):755-66.
38. Wig NN. Hanuman Complex and its Resolution: An Illustration of Psychotherapy from Indian mythology. Indian J Psychiatr. 2004;46(1):25-8.
39. Satyanand D. Recent advances in behavioral therapy. Indian J Psychiatr. 1962;4(2):62-70.
40. Kuruvilla K. Cognitive behaviour therapy yesterday, today & tomorrow. Indian J Psychiatr. 2000;*42*(2):114-24.
41. Chaudhury S, Bakhla AK, Soren S. Ranchi Institute of Neuro-Psychiatry and Allied Sciences: A pioneer in the field of psychiatry in India. Indian J Psychiatr. 2018;60(Suppl 2):S203-11.
42. Selvapandiyan J. Status of cognitive behaviour therapy in India: Pitfalls, limitations and future directions—A systematic review and critical analysis. Asian J Psychiatr. 2019;41:1-4.
43. Row Kavi G, Khanolkar S, Talekar T. Cognitive behavioral therapy in India. In: Terjesen MD, Doyle KA (Eds). Cognitive Behavioral Therapy in a Global Context. Springer Nature Switzerland AG; 2022. pp. 233-55.
44. Kumar N, Gupta P. Cognitive behavioural therapy in India: Adaptations, beliefs and challenges. In: Naeem F, Kingdon D (Eds). Cognitive Behaviour Therapy in Non-Western Cultures; 2012. pp. 61-77.
45. Prasadarao PSDV, Sudhir PM. Clinical psychology in India. J Clin Psychol Med Settings. 2001;8:31-8.
46. Prabhu GG, Shanka R. Clinical Psychology: Coming of Age. In: Agarwal SP, Goel DS, Ichhpujani RL, Salhan RN, Shrivastava S (Eds). Mental Health: An Indian Perspective 1946–2003, New Delhi, Directorate General of Health Services Ministry of Health and Family Welfare; 2004. pp. 123-31.
47. Chakraborty A. External influences on indigenous cultures. World Cultural Psychiatry Research Review. 2007;2(1):3-36.
48. Nandy A. The Intimate Enemy, Loss and Recovery of Self under Colonialism, second edition. New Delhi, Oxford University Press; 2009.
49. Varma VK, Sharan P, Gupta N. Development of an Indian Model of Psychotherapy: Thoughts and Directions for the Future In: Varma VK, Gupta N (Eds). Psychotherapy in Traditional Society: Context Concepts and Practice; 2008. pp. 225-44.

SECTION 1

Inquiring Voices from the Region

2

CHAPTER

The Nature and Extent of Psychotherapy Education during Psychiatry Residency in India

Satish Suhas, Pavithra Jayasankar, Muralidharan Kesavan

ABSTRACT

The chapter "The Nature and Extent of Psychotherapy Education during Psychiatry Residency in India" traces the history of training in psychotherapy in India, the current status of training in psychotherapy in psychiatry residency program and the future directions for psychotherapy training in India. Significant advances have happened in the last few decades in the treatment of mental health disorders including new and advanced psychotherapies. Psychotherapies have also been considered first-line treatment for many mental health disorders. The challenges and opportunities for psychotherapy training in India is also explored in this chapter.

Keywords: Psychotherapy training, Psychiatry residency, India, Postgraduation, Supervision, Therapy

INTRODUCTION

Psychotherapy education within psychiatry residency holds significance, fostering comprehensive patient care and therapeutic proficiency. Psychiatrists integrate psychotherapeutic approaches in their medical practice and, therefore, a structured educational framework is essential. Residents equipped with diverse psychotherapeutic skills can address the psychological aspects of mental disorders. This training helps cultivate empathy, enhancing therapeutic alliance and improves patient outcomes. Moreover, psychotherapy education complements pharmacological interventions, often intersecting with each other, allowing psychiatrists to tailor treatment plans holistically. Ultimately, a well-rounded psychiatry residency incorporating psychotherapy education, not only meets the evolving demands of mental healthcare but also empowers psychiatrists to provide more nuanced, effective, and patient-centered treatment modalities. Psychotherapy training and delivery also has public health implications.[1]

However, challenges in psychotherapy training for psychiatrists are widespread, with many programs needing more comprehensive training standards. Recent shifts in medical education and curriculum present an opportunity to incorporate psychotherapy in psychiatric training. There is a need for academia to cater to this learning need. The strategies to overcome the underdevelopment of psychotherapy training requires the reinforcement of existing expertise and the integration of modern tools and acquisition of new expertise.[2]

HISTORY

The evolution of psychiatry and psychotherapy in India reflects an ethnocentric transformative journey shaped by cultural, social, and medical dynamics. Cultural and religious influences on psychotherapy have been emphasized in literature.[3-6] Traditionally rooted in ancient texts like the Ayurveda, early Indian psychiatry focused on a mind-body connection. The colonial era witnessed Western influences introducing modern psychiatric practices. Postindependence, there was a growing recognition of mental health, culminating in the establishing of mental hospital-based psychiatric institutions. Psychotherapy, deeply embedded in Indian traditions, began gaining recognition alongside pharmacological interventions. Today, a blend of traditional and contemporary approaches characterizes Indian psychiatry.

The Intersection of Philosophy, Mythology, and the Origins of Modern Psychotherapy in India

As Professor Neki had written, in its basic sense, psychotherapy can be defined as an interpersonal method of alleviating distress and therefore by that standard, it has existed since ancient times.[3] Ancient Indian wisdom, rooted in philosophical traditions, harbors psychotherapeutic elements. Practices like Yoga, with its focus on mental wellbeing, and meditation techniques align with modern therapeutic approaches.[7] The concept of mind-body balance in Ayurveda and the emphasis on self-realization contribute to an indigenous foundation for psychotherapeutic principles.[8] Indian epics and scriptures offer psychological insights. The Bhagavad Gita, a dialogue on duty and righteousness, delves into the complexities of the human mind. Characters like Arjuna undergo psychological struggles, providing narrative instances of emotional turmoil and resilience. These ancient texts thus serve as a repository of psychological wisdom with relevance to contemporary therapeutic understanding.[4] Various paradigms including Hanuman complex, Guru-Chela paradigm, Abhyasa paradigm still has its relevance in clinical application.[9] Reports on the formal application of Indian mythology in clinical practice indicate that its utilization has transcended academic or philosophical interest, finding practical application in the real world with increasing cultural acceptability.[10]

Girindrasekhar Bose and Introduction of Western Psychotherapy in India

Girindrasekhar Bose played a pivotal role in the history of psychoanalysis and psychotherapy in India. He emphasized cultural relevance, adapting psychoanalytic techniques to suit Indian sociocultural nuances.

As medical professional he obtained India's first psychology doctorate in 1921. Bose engaged in proto-psychiatry, taught at Calcutta University, and authored psychoanalytic commentaries on classical Indian texts. His work, marked by a blend of Freudian ideas and Indian philosophy, questioned Freudian concepts. Founder of the Indian Psychoanalytic Society, Bose played a pivotal role in bridging the gap between Western psychological paradigms and India's diverse cultural landscape. The history of psychoanalysis in India, through Bose, reveals a unique convergence of Eastern and Western perspectives, challenging established notions and contributing to a distinct psychoanalytic paradigm. This intersection prompts a critical exploration of the 'logic of the Indian psyche' and its dialogues with psychoanalytic thought. Bose's pioneering efforts reflect a rich tapestry of cultural exchange and intellectual evolution in Indian psychotherapy.[11]

The introduction of Western psychotherapy faced initial challenges and resistance in India. Skepticism arose due to cultural disparities and concerns about applicability. Some practitioners were hesitant to adopt foreign methodologies, questioning their relevance to the Indian ethos.[12] Overcoming this resistance required a nuanced understanding of local dynamics and the cultural sensitivity advocated by pioneers like Dr Bose. Despite initial resistance, Western psychotherapy gradually gained acceptance in India. As practitioners recognized its efficacy, a synthesis began, incorporating Western techniques while retaining cultural nuances. There were apprehensions about this arranged union between Western psychotherapy and cultural values of the East as a 'confused and confusing curiosity'.[13] However, with time the adaptability of psychotherapeutic approaches allowed for a harmonious blend, contributing to a more inclusive and diversified mental health landscape in the country.

EVOLUTION OF PSYCHOTHERAPY TRAINING IN INDIA

Emergence of Formal Training Programs

Early initiatives in psychotherapy training were advocated by initial leaders in mental health such as Dr MV Govindaswamy. Recognizing the importance of formal education in psychological interventions, they advocated for specialized training programs. This foresight paved the way for the institutionalization of formal psychotherapy training in postgraduate psychiatry training in India and marked a significant milestone. Institutions like the National Institute of Mental Health and Neurosciences (NIMHANS) played a pivotal role in shaping these programs. As demand grew, academic institutes offering formal training in psychotherapy proliferated.

Psychotherapy Curriculum in Psychiatry Residency

The integration of psychotherapy into psychiatry residency programs reflects a commitment to holistic mental health care. The curriculum encompasses core components and theoretical foundations, emphasizing the multifaceted nature of psychological interventions.

Psychotherapy training in psychiatry residency involves a robust curriculum comprising core components and theoretical foundations. The emphasis is on imparting essential skills, understanding diverse therapeutic modalities, and grounding practitioners in evidence-based practices to address the complexities of mental health. To foster versatility, the curriculum integrates diverse psychotherapeutic approaches. Cognitive-behavioral therapy, psychodynamic interventions, and humanistic approaches are harmoniously included. This integration equips mental health professionals with a nuanced understanding, enabling them to tailor interventions to individual needs.

The integration of psychoanalytic thought alongside other approaches becomes pivotal for stabilizing trainees facing roadblocks, enhancing their skills in navigating challenges, particularly with difficult-to-treat patients in tertiary settings. Initial training programs focused on humanistic and psychoanalytical/psychodynamic forms of psychotherapy. Whereas, the psychotherapy training has now evolved over the past 5 decades to incorporate newer schools of psychotherapy including cognitive behavioral therapy, specialized forms of behavioral therapy and newer transdiagnostic therapies such as mindfulness-based therapy. A growing trend in contemporary therapeutic practice involves adopting a client-centered approach while affording trainees the flexibility to integrate components from diverse therapeutic schools. This results in an emerging preference for an eclectic approach to therapy.

CASE STUDY: NIMHANS PSYCHOTHERAPY TRAINING PROGRAM

Psychotherapy training has been an integral part of the NIMHANS for over four decades, evolving into a flagship program within the Department of Psychiatry. This retrospective explores the inception, structural changes, and advancements in the psychotherapy training program at NIMHANS.

Pioneering Initiatives

In the late seventies, when formal psychotherapy training was lacking at NIMHANS, Professor C Shamasundar initiated pilot programs in 1978. These included weekly exercises in psychodynamics of interviewing, ward-group meetings, and self-experience groups. These endeavors aimed to stimulate awareness and interest in psychotherapy among faculty and psychiatry residents. The initial exercises led to a shift in the institutional atmosphere, prompting more residents to seek individual supervision in psychotherapy. Consequently, a formal psychotherapy training program for psychiatry residents was inaugurated in August 1983. They met weekly to formulate, implement, and monitor the program. The focus was on promoting dynamic psychotherapy, with residents required to complete a minimum of 25 supervised sessions per year.

Shaping the Curriculum and Training Philosophy

Supervisor competence is pivotal in psychotherapy training, requiring specific training for knowledge, skills, and attitudes. Supervisors serve as role models, protect the patient's interests, and act as gatekeepers, ensuring that the residents (and supervisees) meet competence standards. They strive for competence in psychotherapy services, possess up-to-date knowledge, and seek formal education to maintain competence in supervision. Coordination with professionals involved in supervisee education, diversity competence, and ethical use of technology are integral aspects of supervisor responsibility, highlighting the need for continuous education and adherence to ethical standards in the evolving landscape of psychological supervision. This underscores the importance of a psychotherapy training curriculum. Additionally, the curriculum evolves periodically, thus reflecting a dynamic training philosophy, aligning with contemporary mental health needs and evidence-based medicine. Any curriculum should be shaped by pioneers, it encompasses theoretical foundations, skill development, and an integrative approach that acknowledges the cultural context of psychotherapy practice.

Different Phases of Training

The training program consisted of distinct phases detailed elsewhere:[14]

- *Preparation:* New residents received introductory reading lists and lectures on the training program's description and principles of psychotherapy.
- *Clarification:* Supervisors engaged residents in discussions to address theoretical and practical issues, easing anxieties, misunderstandings, and doubts.
- *Interview exercises:* Residents familiarized themselves with psychodynamics through rotations, presenting interview sessions for group discussions.
- *Supervision of psychotherapy:* Individual and group supervision became integral, focusing on refining interview skills, identifying core conflicts, and formulating practical therapeutic objectives. The compulsory weekly

supervision of psychotherapy student groups not only guarantees that residents learn from their individual experiences but also facilitates learning through the collective experiences of their peers. The supervisors' group, initially comprising 11 members, has now expanded to over 40, reflecting the program's growth. Noteworthy is the incorporation of behavioral therapy, family therapy, mindfulness-based therapy, dialectical behavioral therapy, grief therapy, motivation enhancement therapy, brief psychodynamic therapy to the already existing training in psychodynamic therapy, cognitive behavioral therapy, and supportive psychotherapies. This helps in fostering an eclectic approach to training. Additionally, technological integration, particularly during the COVID-19 pandemic, has revolutionized the training landscape. The Psychotherapy Coordination Committee oversees program supervision and activities.

The initial psychotherapy supervision program included the following components:

- *Individual and group supervision:* Initially limited to second-year residents, individual supervision involved weekly meetings between each resident and their assigned supervisor. From September 1984 onwards, group supervision became mandatory for all residents. Each supervisor led a group of 5 to 7 residents in weekly sessions.
- *Supervisory sessions:* Residents presented psychotherapy material, emphasizing the refinement of skills, identification of core conflicts, and the formulation of practical therapeutic objectives. Some sessions involve reading transcripts or audio/video recordings of the therapy sessions (that is reviewed in the group with the patients consent).
- *Assessment:* The resident's performance in psychotherapy contributed to internal assessment. Initial and final assessments, coupled with supervisor evaluations, were conducted to gauge adherence to the program, participation, and therapeutic functioning.
- *Theoretical reinforcement:* Second-year residents were exposed to tutorials on various psychotherapy schools and are encouraged to take up therapy for complex clinical presentations.

Phases of Current Psychotherapy Supervision and Training at NIMHANS during Postgraduate Psychiatry Residency

NIMHANS' psychotherapy training unfolds in phases, fostering a comprehensive skill set among residents.

Early Phase: Basic Skills and Communication Skills Development

The program prioritizes communication skills as foundational. Residents undergo systematic training to enhance verbal and nonverbal communication skills, helpful responses, and empathic communication, vital for establishing therapeutic alliances. This phase also includes education about desirable therapist qualities and conscious effort to imbibe the same in practice. These skills will help forge the all-important therapeutic relationship that is essential for psychotherapy. These are developed through the Rogerian principles of empathy, genuineness, integrity, hopefulness, trust in ability of the patient to get well, and unconditional positive regard. This coupled with reflection and self-monitoring of one's therapeutic behavior are fundamental skills in the therapist. In this phase, there is a consolidation of group dynamics and there is a degree of freedom that the supervisee develops enabling them to freely exchange ideas, reflect and be open to continuous process of learning. In the initial stages, it is imperative to familiarize oneself with crucial elements of documentation pertaining to therapy session records. Additionally, it is essential to establish collaborative empiricism with the patient, involving them in the process of defining overarching therapeutic goals and formulating specific session objectives. This early phase lays the foundation for a comprehensive and effective therapeutic journey.

Middle Phase: Core Supervision

During this phase, the supervisor discusses cases seen by the supervisees for therapy. Hands-on therapeutic interview exercises deepen practical competencies. Residents engage in simulated sessions, refining their abilities to apply diverse therapeutic modalities. There could be innovative ways of managing these exercises through demonstrations by supervisors, role-play within the group, or even in-person sessions with the patient. This middle phase is a period where supervisees gain insights into transference, countertransference, and overcoming various challenges during the psychotherapeutic process.

Continuation Phase: Theoretical Reinforcement and Academic Training

Theoretical foundations receive emphasis through academic training. Residents gain in-depth knowledge of psychotherapeutic approaches, ensuring a robust theoretical framework informs their practice. These reinforcements and trainings can be through access to recommended reading, e-resources, case conferences, grand-rounds, continuing-medical education programs, academic conferences. NIMHANS adapts to technological advancements, integrating modern tools into psychotherapy training. This approach aligns with evolving healthcare landscapes, preparing residents for contemporary challenges. One of the achievements of the institute, led by the Department of Clinical Psychology was to develop the guidelines for telepsychotherapy services in 2020 during the COVID-19 pandemic,[15] thereby ensuring uninterrupted provision of psychotherapy to the patients in need.

Termination Phase

Here, the supervisee is trained to handle aspects related to therapy termination and empowerment of the supervisee themselves become navigators of the therapeutic processes and ultimately start developing self-assurance as a psychotherapist. In the larger ambit of learning, the supervisee realizes that the termination phase in essence is the completion of the preparatory phase and an acquisition of a metaphorical license for life-long learning in psychotherapy.

Supervision and Assessment

Supervision and assessment play pivotal roles, ensuring quality and skill enhancement. Assessment, evaluation, and feedback form integral aspects of supervision, yet their infrequent provision poses challenges in gatekeeping and informing supervisees about competency development. Ideally, these processes occur within a collaborative relationship, anchored in the supervisee's competency development. Supervisors monitor and provide feedback on performance through live observation or recorded sessions, acknowledging the limitations of self-report. Feedback is delivered directly, clearly, and timely, considering power differentials, cultural diversity, and supervisee developmental levels. Supervisors recognize the value of supervisee self-assessment, incorporating it into the evaluation process. They also seek regular feedback from supervisees and others, utilizing it to enhance their supervisory competence.

Role of Supervisors and Coordination

Experienced supervisors play a crucial role, guiding residents through their psychotherapeutic journey. Coordination between supervisors ensures a cohesive and effective training experience.

Evaluation Methods and Feedback Mechanisms

NIMHANS employs diverse evaluation methods, including case presentations and assessments. Feedback mechanisms are structured, fostering continuous improvement and personalized development plans. Each year, academic awards for excellence in psychotherapy are conferred upon students following a comprehensive assessment. This evaluation involves cumulative scoring, encompassing marks assigned by the therapy supervisor, evaluations of case records, and a psychotherapy viva examination conducted by two independent psychiatry faculty members from the department.

Calendar of Psychotherapy Training

Residents are allocated to supervisors early in their tenure, with a comprehensive communication skills workshop initiating their residency. Regular meetings with supervisors, theoretical lectures, and practical training sessions lead to a final examination in the 32nd month of the training period out of 36 months of postgraduate training. The program has evolved to address contemporary challenges and opportunities, such as the integration of telepsychotherapy. The training calendar underscores strategic planning and adaptability.

Allocation to Supervisors and Resident Involvement

Residents are strategically allocated to supervisors, considering their individual learning needs. Active resident involvement in the process fosters a sense of ownership. Although personal apprenticeship is ideal, group psychotherapy supervision is more pragmatic.

Weekly Training Sessions and Examination Processes

Weekly training sessions form a consistent rhythm, complemented by examination processes that gauge residents' grasp of theoretical concepts and practical applications.

Exposure to Specialized Forms of Therapy

NIMHANS residents undergo specialized training in behavioral therapy through a formal 1 month posting in the Behavioral Therapy Unit, complemented by an additional month dedicated to training in family therapy. Furthermore, residents receive comprehensive training in various therapeutic modalities, including child and adolescent psychiatry therapy, therapy for the elderly, and motivation enhancement therapy for individuals with substance use disorders. These multifaceted training experiences occur during rotations in specialty clinics and individual subspecialties.

Evolution and Adaptability Over the Years

NIMHANS' psychotherapy training program has evolved over the years, staying adaptable to emerging trends. Continuous refinement ensures alignment with evolving psychotherapeutic paradigms, contributing to its enduring success. Comparing the program's status in 1993 to 2020 reveals significant growth in the number of supervisors, technological advancements, and the integration of diverse therapeutic modalities. While the core principles persist, the program has adapted to the changing landscape of psychotherapy practice.

Psychotherapy Supervision in the Era of Consumer Protection and Mental Healthcare Act of 2017

Ethics, legal, and regulatory considerations are paramount in clinical supervision, ensuring the highest standards of professional conduct and protecting the wellbeing of clients and patients. Improper or inadequate supervision can lead to disciplinary actions by licensing boards. Supervisors model ethical behavior, by adhering to standard ethical guidelines, professional organizations' guidelines, and relevant laws and regulations. They foster supervisees' ethical and legal acculturation, integrating ethics into professional behavior.

The primary ethical and legal obligation of supervisors is to protect the welfare of the client/patient. Balancing this with the secondary responsibility of increasing supervisee competence, supervisors ensure supervisees understand their responsibilities regarding clinical performance. Serving as gatekeepers to the profession, supervisors assess supervisees' suitability to enter and remain in the field, advancing them based on competencies or addressing competency problems following explicit organizational plans.

Supervisors provide clear information about supervision expectations through a written supervisory contract, specifying roles, tasks, and responsibilities. The contract includes elements such as the content, method, and context of supervision, highest duties of the supervisor, roles and expectations of both parties, evaluation criteria, and processes for ethical problem-solving. Accurate and timely documentation of supervisee performance is maintained to track competency and professional development, supporting accountability and adherence to ethical standards.

International Collaborations

The inaugural digital conference, "Psychotherapy across epochs and methods," was held on September 11th and 12th, 2020, marked a significant collaboration between two esteemed institutions: The NIMHANS in India and the Tavistock and Portman, National Health Service (NHS) Foundation Trust in the UK. Renowned for their contributions to psychotherapy training and service provision, the conference covered diverse themes, incorporating participant feedback. The discussions delved into the evolving role of technology in both psychotherapy services and training, addressing current and future considerations. The conference was attended discussions spanned a broad spectrum, beginning with an exploration of psychotherapy training in India and extending to the UK. Delving into therapeutic nuances, topics include internalizations in child sexual abuse therapy, trauma approaches, and tailored therapies for externalizing behavior spectrum difficulties and personality disorders, and interventions for patients with physical symptoms. Technology's role in psychotherapy, from self-care to professional interventions, and the prospects and challenges of telepsychotherapy in psychiatry training, provided contemporary insights. The collective knowledge and insights were discussed in a panel discussion, offering varied perspectives and snippets on psychotherapy.[16]

PSYCHOTHERAPY TRAINING ACROSS INDIA

Overview of Psychotherapy Training in Different Institutions

Our exploration of psychotherapy training for psychiatry postgraduates in various Indian institutes draws from significant literature. It is tabulated as follows:

Study title	*Authors*	*Type of study*	*Major findings*
Training postgraduate students of psychiatry in psychotherapy at Bombay[17]	LP Shah	Narrative review	Highlights the absence of structured psychotherapy training program in colleges in Bombay
Task force guidelines for postgraduate psychiatry training in India[18]	Issac M, et al.	Survey	56.1% colleges mandate psychotherapy training, though specific training program are not available
An experiment in psychotherapy training. Indian Journal of Psychiatry[19]	Tharyan A	Intervention study	Feasibility of group supervision in psychotherapy training
Evaluation of psychiatry training in India: A survey of young psychiatrists under the aegis of research, education, and training foundation of Indian Psychiatric Society[20]	Grover S, et al.	Survey	Psychotherapy training quality was rated poor by 34.8% survey participants
Are we meeting training needs? Training and its influence on the practice of child psychiatry and psychotherapy[21]	Kishore AN et al.	Survey	Around 35% psychiatrists report no psychotherapy training during their postgraduation

Challenges and Opportunities

Identifying Gaps in Psychotherapy Education

While the Medical Council of India (MCI), the erstwhile name for the National Medical Commission, outlines psychotherapy training in its curriculum, the absence of a unified program nationwide stems from various factors, as outlined by existing literature.[17] Trainer-related issues encompass infrequent psychotherapy use, inadequate trainer training, and trainers' inability to stimulate learning. Student-related challenges involve a lack of interest, temperamental unsuitability, and an overemphasis on the biological model of mental illness. Milieu-related factors include patient overcrowding, limited teaching hours, a shortage of skilled trainers and equipment, and a migratory patient population. Addressing these gaps is imperative for devising a comprehensive psychotherapy training module for postgraduates in training institutes.

Standardization of Curricula and Guidelines

While MCI emphasizes the performance of behavior and family therapy, along with assisting experts in interpersonal therapy at the end of psychiatry postgraduate training, formal mandates for psychotherapy training and assessments are lacking in the curriculum.[22] Recognizing the significance of psychotherapy in clinical practice, it is crucial to integrate it as a compulsory component in postgraduate training. The Indian Psychiatric Society (IPS) task force in 2013 proposed two approaches for psychotherapy tutorials, recommending weekly supervision in large departments and case conferences in smaller ones, with a minimum of 50 hours of supervised psychotherapy and case submission as part of internal assessment.[18] However, existing evidence highlights heterogeneity in psychotherapy training across centers, underscoring the need for standardized curricula and guidelines.[23] Therefore, at the MCI level, there is a pressing need to mandate psychotherapy training in the postgraduate curriculum, while IPS, at the organizational level, should conduct Continuing Medical Education (CME) focusing on psychotherapies and hands-on training for young psychiatrists. At the institute/college level, mandatory 50-hour supervised psychotherapy and case submission in the final year should be implemented.

Standardization also requires formal training for supervisors too. At least one or more faculty from an institute/college should undergo formal training in psychotherapy from a central agency (e.g., IPS) who can then become master trainer to develop the psychotherapy program in their respective colleges.

Incorporating Technological Advancements

Leveraging technological advancements, incorporating technology in psychotherapy training emerges as a viable avenue. Traditional clinical supervision, relying on verbal reports or session recordings for feedback, often faces limitations due to time and resource constraints, resulting in a lack of detailed case discussions. Computational technologies offer a solution, with clinical support tools capable of providing automated feedback to counselors based on session audio, assessing counselor empathy, specific skills, and emotional arousal at the utterance level. While these technologies have the potential to enhance and streamline psychotherapy interactions, practical concerns such as data collection, dissemination, and apprehensions about observation may impact their widespread implementation in training.[24-27]

Emerging Directions and Recommendations

Changing Landscape of Psychotherapy Education

Psychotherapy education has evolved through different stages, incorporating various schools of therapy, with over 450 therapy models identified in recent research. LSS. Manickam's review on "Psychotherapy in India" divides its history into three phases: (1) An initial phase with psychoanalytical concepts, (2) A middle phase embracing psychodynamic, humanistic, and existential concepts, and (3) A current phase characterized by an eclectic and integrative stance.[28] The debate over the applicability of Western psychotherapy to the Indian population dates to the 1950s, with many Indian psychiatrists noting challenges in its adaptability. Verma identified seven distinct features of the Indian population that may impede the efficacy of psychotherapy, including dependence/interdependence, lack of psychological sophistication, and social distance between doctor and patient.[29,30]

Despite these concerns, Shamasundar and Rao practiced psychotherapy and tested its applicability in the Indian context. Globalization, increased education, heightened awareness of human rights, and widespread electronic media use, even in rural areas, have contributed to growing acceptance of psychotherapy in India. Consequently, psychotherapy education must consider these changing attitudes, considering the sociocultural milieu and regional variations.[28-33]

Advancing Formalized Training Programs

The current state of psychotherapy training exhibits significant variation, ranging from mandatory programs in some institutes to the absence of training in others. To enhance postgraduate psychotherapy training, established systems within the education sector[34] can be integrated, emphasizing uniformity in content, formalized training modules, and objective assessments. It is essential to devise mechanisms for consistently incorporating the latest knowledge and updating the curriculum to align with evolving social, economic, and technological landscapes.

Accreditation bodies, particularly the MCI, hold a crucial role in advancing training programs by regularly revising the curriculum. Additionally, the implementation of periodic CME sessions, workshops, and student exchange programs focused on psychotherapy can provide students nationwide with comprehensive training opportunities in this field. Recently, a psychotherapy subcommittee has been established by the IPS.[35] We hope that this subcommittee will conduct nation-wide training programs in psychotherapy which can cater to psychiatry postgraduates across the country.

Technological Integration and Innovation

Expanding Telepsychotherapy and E-learning

COVID-19 pandemic has dramatically changed the psychotherapy practices around the world. It has shifted from predominantly face to face settings to online settings since the beginning of pandemic.[36] The ethical and legal guidelines in telepsychotherapy in India was released in April 2020.[37] Apart from teletherapy, these digital platforms can also be used to conduct e-workshops and online CMEs which would potentially increase the audience base and wide outreach to students across the country. However, standardization of training and certification by regulatory bodies is also important to ensure the quality of training.

Collaboration and Networking

World Health Organization (WHO) in collaboration with World Psychiatric Association (WPA)[38] published an overview of psychiatric education and training across the world and revealed a marked variability in training and regional variation. To improve standards and exchange of knowledge, networking with other institutes across the world becomes crucial. Such international collaborations can occur in the form of conferences, workshops, student exchange programs, research collaboration and so on. Regulatory bodies such as MCI and WHO can also facilitate such collaborations to develop the standards of medical education and to improve the quality of health care.

Ensuring Quality and Competence

Validation of Psychotherapeutic Training

There are many difficulties related to the evaluation of standards of psychotherapy training. However, with technological advancements and blooming rise of various platforms to provide training, it becomes essential to validate the training programs. The tripartite model which includes didactic training, supervision and personal psychotherapy has been the most acknowledged model of clinical training.[39] The validation in psychotherapy training should occur at structure (module) level, trainer (supervisors) level and at regulatory level. Also there should be a broad overview in the curriculum about the contents and methods of psychotherapy training. In addition to this, evaluation of these training programs and training of supervisors should occur in a periodic basis.

Standards for Ethical Practice and Patient Care

The three most important issues for the best ethical practice include positive ethics, risk management and defensive practice.[40] Positive ethics focusses on the constant efforts made by the therapist for achieving the best possible ethical standards. Risk management focusses on reducing the risks for the therapist in the form of complaints to the ethics bodies or malpractice claims. Defensive practice focusses on direct protection of the therapist and involves decision making based on reducing the possibility of adverse outcomes for the therapist. Based on these three principles, the ethical and legal guidelines for psychotherapy[41] focuses on competence and responsibilities of a therapist, therapeutic contract, confidentiality, documentation, boundaries, self-disclosure, professional negligence, termination, and post-termination issues. It is the responsibility of therapist to be aware of the ethical and legal principles involved in psychotherapy. Hence, understanding these ethical principles should be imparted in the psychotherapy training program.

CONCLUSION

Psychotherapy forms integral form of clinical service delivery for the effective management of psychiatric disorders. Over the years, different schools of psychotherapy have emerged and various modalities (in person, teletherapy) have been in use. To achieve good quality of psychotherapy training in India, efforts must be taken at various levels from trainee level to regulatory bodies level. A standardized uniform training module should be devised for all the postgraduates. Regular CMEs and workshops for students and trainers should be conducted to improve the standard of care. The IPS and central institutes can take the instrumental lead in modelling of psychotherapy training and standardization of the psychotherapy training curriculum.

REFERENCES

1. Sriram TG. Psychotherapy in developing countries: a public health perspective. Indian J Psychiatry. 1990;32(2):138-44.

2. Holmes J, Mizen S, Jacobs C. Psychotherapy training for psychiatrists: UK and global perspectives. International Review of Psychiatry. 2007;19(1):93-100.
3. Neki JS. Psychotherapy in India: Past, Present, and Future. APT. 1975;29(1):92-100.
4. Reddy MS. Psychotherapy–Insights from Bhagavad Gita. Indian J Psychol Med. 2012;34(1):100-4.
5. Hoch EM. Experiences with psychotherapy training in India. Psychother Psychosom. 2010;53(1–4):14-20.
6. Shamasundar C. Some personal reflections relating to psychotherapy. Indian J Psychiatry. 2008;50(4):301-4.
7. Caplan M, Portillo A, Seely L. Yoga psychotherapy: The integration of western psychological theory and ancient yogic wisdom. J Transpersonal Psychol. 2013;45(2):139-58.
8. Behere PB, Das A, Yadav R, Behere AP. Ayurvedic concepts related to psychotherapy. Indian J Psychiatry. 2013;55(Suppl 2):S310-4.
9. Van Hoecke G. Paradigms in Indian psychotherapy: Applicability in a Western approach. Mental Health, Religion & Culture. 2006;9(02):119-25.
10. Shamasundar C. Therapeutic wisdom in Indian mythology. Am J Psychother. 1993;47(3):443-50.
11. Dhar A. Girindrasekhar Bose and the History of Psychoanalysis in India. Indian J History Science. 2018;534:T198-T204. [online] Available from https://www.academia.edu/38858598/Girindrasekhar_Bose_and_the_History_of_Psychoanalysis_in_India [Last accessed December, 2023].
12. Varma VK. Present state of psychotherapy in India. Indian J Psychiatry. 1982;24(3):209-26.
13. Ratna L. Psychotherapeutic Processes: Proceedings of the Seminar held at NIMHANS in October 1978. Edited by Kapur M, Murthy VN, Sathyavathi K and Kapur RL Bangalore, India: National Institute of Mental Health and Neuro Sciences. 1979. Pp 159.
14. Shamasundar C, Verghese M, Raguram R, Jain S, Girimaji S, Seshadri S, et al. Psychotherapy programme for psychiatry residents at NIMHANS-1. A descriptive account. Indian J Psychiatry. 1993;35(4):215-7.
15. NIMHANS D of CP. Guidelines for tele-psychotherapy services. [online] Available from https://nimhans.ac.in/wp-content/uploads/2020/04/Guidelines-for-Telepsychotherapy-Services-17.4.2020.pdf [Last accessed December, 2023].
16. Suhas S, Chithra NK, Nair S, Huddar S, Naik SS, SL, et al. Psychotherapy across epochs and methods NIMHANS – TAVISTOCK Psychotherapy conference. Asian J Psychiatry. 2021;56:102459.
17. Kapur, M, Shamasundar C, Bhatti RS. Psychotherapy Training in India. Bangalore: NIMHANS, 1996.
18. Issac M, Murthy P, Sidana A, Sharma P, Ghosal M, Subodh BN. Task force guidelines for postgraduate psychiatry training in India. Indian Psychiatric Society; 2013.
19. Tharyan A. An experiment in psychotherapy training. Indian J Psychiatry. 2000;42(2):142.
20. Grover S, Sahoo S, Srinivas B, Tripathi A, Avasthi A. Evaluation of psychiatry training in India: A survey of young psychiatrists under the aegis of research, education, and training foundation of Indian Psychiatric Society. Indian J Psychiatry. 2018;60(4):445.

21. Kishore ANR, Shaji KS, Praveenlal K. Revalidation: Are we meeting training needs? Training and its influence on the practice of child psychiatry and psychotherapy. Indian J Psychol Med. 2010;32(1):3-6.
22. Medical Council of India. Guidelines for competency-based postgraduate training programs for MD psychiatry; 2002.
23. Kakunje A, Punnoose VP, Ponnusamy KP, Mysore AV, Daniel SJ. Revisiting postgraduate (PG) psychiatry training in India. Indian J Psychol Med. 2019;41(4):380-7.
24. Amerikaner M, Rose T. Direct observation of psychology supervisees' clinical work: A snapshot of current practice. The Clinical Supervisor. 2012;31(1):61-80.
25. Gibson J, Gray G, Hirsch T, Imel ZE, Narayanan SS, Atkins DC. Developing an automated report card for addiction counseling: The counselor observer ratings expert for MI (CORE-MI). Paper presented at the Computer Human Interaction. Mental Health Workshop; San Jose, CA, USA. 2016. pp. 1-4.
26. Imel ZE, Caperton DD, Tanana M, Atkins DC. Technology-enhanced human interaction in psychotherapy. J Couns Psychol. 2017;64(4):385.
27. Hirsch T, Merced K, Imel Z, Narayanan S, Atkins D. Designing Contestability: Interaction Design, Machine Learning, and Mental Health. DIS (Des Interact Syst Conf). 2017;2017:95-99.
28. Manickam LS. Psychotherapy in India. Indian journal of psychiatry. 2010;52(Suppl1): S366-70.
29. Varma VK. Present state of psychotherapy in India. Indian J Psychiatry. 1982;24(3):209.
30. Shamasundar C. Some personal reflections relating to psychotherapy. Indian J Psychiatry. 2008;50(4):301.
31. Neki JS. Confidentiality, secrecy, and privacy in psychotherapy: Sociodynamic considerations. Indian J Psychiatry. 1992;34(3):171.
32. Surya NC, Jayaram SS. Some Basic Considerations in the practice of Psychotherapy in the Indian Setting. Indian J Psychiatry. 1964;6(3):153-6.
33. Boss M. The role of psychotherapy in schizophrenia. Indian J Psychiatry. 1958;1(1):4-12.
34. Sharma S. Postgraduate training in psychiatry in India. Indian J Psychiatry. 2010;52(Suppl1):S89-94.
35. Indian Psychiatric Society. IPS Sub-Committees, Specialty Sections, Task Forces, Commissions & Tribunal [Internet]. 2023 [cited 2023 Dec 30]; Available from https://indianpsychiatricsociety.org/wp-content/uploads/2023/03/IPS-Committees-2023-2024-F1.pdf.
36. Tajan N, Devès M, Potier R. Tele-psychotherapy during the COVID-19 pandemic: a mini-review. Front Psychiatry. 2023;14:1060961.
37. Bhola P, Poornima MN. Guidelines for Tele-Psychotherapy Services. Ver. 1. 2020 Bengaluru National Institute of Mental Health and Neuro Sciences (NIMHANS).
38. Saxena S. Atlas: Psychiatric education and training across the world 2005. World Health Organization; 2005
39. Gurman AS, Razin AM. Effective psychotherapy: A Handbook of Research; 1977.
40. Barnett JE. Positive ethics, risk management, and defensive practice. Md Psychol. 2007; 53:30-1.
41. Avasthi A, Grover S, Nischal A. Ethical and legal issues in psychotherapy. Indian J Psychiatry. 2022;64(Suppl 1):S47.

3 CHAPTER

Current State of Psychotherapeutic and Psychoanalytic Practice in India

Gagan Hans, Sumegha Mittal

ABSTRACT

In India, the practice of psychotherapy is still in its early stages of development. The growth of psychotherapy in India is significantly influenced by various deep rooted cultural factors in society. However, there has been a noticeable improvement in people's awareness and willingness to seek therapy over the past decade. Although research on the adaptation of psychotherapy to the Indian cultural context is limited, efforts are being made to effectively integrate psychotherapy within the cultural parameters. This chapter explores strategies for adapting psychological therapies to the general clinical population. Currently very limited research is conducted in this field and further research is needed to gain a deeper understanding of how psychological interventions can be successfully implemented in the Indian context. Through ongoing efforts, it is hoped that practice of psychotherapy is expected to witness a significant increase in India.

Keywords: Psychotherapy, Psychotherapy training, Cognitive behavior therapy, India

INTRODUCTION AND BRIEF HISTORICAL CONSIDERATIONS

Since its introduction to India, psychological concepts have faced resistance from scholars and general population as these have been perceived as foreign to the culture of India. India is a secular country with variety of traditions and beliefs. In India, religion and spirituality have always played an integral role in matters concerning the psychological health. Overtime, some efforts have been made to cultivate Indian philosophies and cultural paradigm in the practices of psychoanalysis and psychotherapy in the country.

The origins of psychotherapy in India are somewhat elusive, lacking definitive historical milestones. Nonetheless, according to Indian mythology and ancient scriptures, some related forms of psychotherapeutic practices have always existed in the country for centuries. India being the birthplace of four major religions of the world, it is no surprise that religious concepts and teachings including those from ancient scriptures, have seamlessly woven themselves into the fabric of 'psychotherapeutic' process.

References to counseling in ancient times can be found in various religious and philosophical texts like the Vedas and the Bhagavad Gita. The Bhagavad Gita, the holy book could be the first example of actual "live one to one counseling", with Lord Krishna explaining the philosophy of life to

Arjuna, during the epic war, Mahabharata. The Vedas focus on spiritual and emotional growth of an individual and helps to achieve good psychological health. Psychodynamic psychotherapy, cognitive-behavioral therapy (CBT), mindfulness, grief therapy, interpersonal therapy (IPT), addiction therapy, and supportive psychotherapy have similarities with Bhagavad Gita, an ancient Indian scripture *(Bhatia et al., 2013).*

The practice of psychotherapy has several challenges in India when compared with west. To mention a few: Indian population has different psychological mindedness than their western counterparts, there is a strong influence of sociocultural and religious beliefs, the concept of personal responsibility and accountability varies, the concept of karma is deep rooted and the issues surrounding confidentiality differ from western practices, all of which potentially affects the therapeutic relationship. The composition of the society drastically changed with urbanization and industrialization leading to increased rural to urban migration and the society was turned from a collectivistic society to individualistic in nature. These impacts of industrialization, migration, social issues on mental health were investigated and newer therapies like behavior therapies, cognitive and third wave therapies paved their ways and became more popular *(Verma SK, 1998).*

NEED OF PSYCHOTHERAPY AND MENTAL HEALTH SERVICES IN INDIA

According to the World Health Organization (WHO), mental and behavioral disorders are responsible for approximately 13% of the worldwide burden of disorders *(World Mental Health Report,* 2022*)*. However, this figure may be an underestimate, given the interconnectedness of mental illness with other socioeconomic factors, particularly in low- and middle-income countries (LMICs), which bear nearly three quarters of the global burden of mental and behavioral disorders. In India, an estimated 197.3 million individuals are affected by mental disorders.

In the context of India, mental health and substance use disorders have a significant impact on the well-being of individuals. These disorders are the primary cause of nonfatal burden of disease, measured as Years Lost to Disability (YLD), and the fifth leading cause of increased burden of Disability Adjusted Life Years (DALYs). Among the group of mental health and substance use disorders, depressive and anxiety disorders contribute the most to DALYs and YLDs. It is estimated that more than 75% of mental health issues remain unaddressed. In the field of psychiatry in India, there is a notable lack of utilization of psychosocial treatments *('The Burden of Mental Disorders across the States of India,' 2020).*

A survey conducted in 1973 by Varma and Ghosh revealed that only 17% of Indian Psychiatric Society Fellows reported using any form of psychological treatment. Although the number of psychiatrists in India has increased since then, it is unlikely that the percentage of those employing psychological methods has significantly changed. This limited adoption of psychosocial treatments can also be seen in the research published in the Indian Journal of Psychiatry (IJP), which dedicates only about 2% of its papers to this area compared to 16% in the British Journal of Psychiatry *(Kuruvilla, 2010)*.

Providing mental health services for this large population is undeniably a challenging task. This challenge is further compounded by limited financial resources, the coexistence of diverse and conflicting healing traditions, a shortage of mental health professionals, the "brain drain" phenomenon, and the stigma associated with seeking assistance for mental health issues. Insufficient budgeting and underutilization of funds are hindering mental health service development in India. The 2021–2022 union budget (712.69 billion INR) allocated only 5.97 billion INR to mental health (Union Budget for Mental Health 2023–2024). Moreover, there is a substantial treatment gap in both developed and developing nations, with a vast majority of patients in LMICs lacking access to mental and behavioral disorder treatment facilities. There is shortage of mental health professionals in India. There are only two mental health workers and 0.3 psychiatrists per 100,000 population. This scarcity needs to be addressed and the problem is exacerbated by factors like urban concentration and brain drain of the mental health professionals *(Mental Health Atlas 2017 Country Profile,)*.

Psychotherapy also helps to reduce perceived stigma amongst patients with mental health problems by providing them a safe space to discuss about their concerns and seek help. There is a growing awareness of importance of mental health in India and in turn increased demand for psychotherapy services as people seek professional support for their mental wellbeing. The need for psychotherapy in India is driven by increasing recognition of mental health issues, stigma reduction, a response to various social, cultural and lifestyle challenges. Access to professional mental health support through psychotherapy is essential for wellbeing of individuals and communities in India.

BARRIERS TO ESTABLISH PSYCHOTHERAPY AS FIRST-LINE TREATMENT IN INDIA

In India, mental health conditions are mostly neglected and not considered disorders unlike physical ailments. There is a general perception that these conditions improve on their own without any active intervention. Help is sought for these problems only at later stages. People first seek help from the family, religious institutes, astrologer, or faith healers. Psychological disturbances may be considered a sign of weakness at times especially by male members of the society and they seldom seek treatment. Stigma is another important factor in Indian society for not seeking treatment. In the country, although the burden of mental disorders is very high, but the awareness about the availability of treatment is very limited. Those who seek treatment want a quick relief in their symptoms, hence they prefer pharmacological treatment over psychotherapy. Psychotherapy is considered as time-consuming requiring prolonged engagement with the therapist. Psychotherapy is equated with counseling and patients expect to tell their problems to the therapist and get some advice on the same. Moreover, therapy sessions are also expensive compared to pharmacotherapy *(Cognitive Behavioral Therapy in a Global Context | Springer Link,* n.d.*)*.

PSYCHOTHERAPY CONCEPTS IN INDIA

The traditional model of "guru-chela" relationship in Indian culture has stood the test of time as in this unique concept of psychotherapy, the teacher serves as a mentor and counselor and plays a pivotal role in guiding the student through the critical decisions and fostering profound insights in all the domains of life *(Neki, 1975)*. The relationship can be seen as an early form of psychotherapy, gradually evolving to encompass family therapy, and occasionally involving family members in the counseling sessions. Additionally, supportive therapy found its place alongside other psychotherapeutic approaches. There is a significant emphasis on interdependency, resulting in a heightened dependency of client on the therapist or counselor. The religious and spiritual teaching have always emphasized on focusing and correcting one's own thought processes, beliefs, and feelings instead of holding external situations and factors responsible for their psychological disturbances. In psychodynamic psychotherapy, the Gita's concept of the three *gunas (tamas, rajas, and sattva)* is compared to Freud's structural theory of the id, ego, and superego. Both theories emphasize the resolution of conflicts and the promotion of adaptation. The Gita also discusses the role of the senses and the mind in relation to psychoanalytic concepts.

CBT and the Gita share commonalities in addressing cognitive distortions and promoting behavioral change. In Gita, different cognitive distortions like catastrophizing the future and personalization, in which is excessively worrying about the future and holding himself guilty. Lord Krishna addresses and corrects these by explaining using the principle of karma and that everything in this world takes their natural course of action and that Arjuna is misunderstanding by holding himself responsible for all the actions. Lord Krishna resolves Arjuna's conflict by telling him that *atman* is eternal, and he will not be held responsible for the demise of his cousins. The Gita's principles of detachment, *karma yoga* (action without attachment), and mindfulness align with CBT techniques such as challenging irrational thoughts and promoting present-moment awareness. The Gita's teachings can be integrated into supportive psychotherapy by providing pragmatic guidance, reframing perceptions, and promoting adaptive behaviors *(Bhatia et al., 2013)*.

Later when behavior therapy, cognitive therapy, and other therapies paved their way in west slowly they were also introduced in India and were adapted according to Indian culture. In India, there is a preference for a 'holistic' approach to therapy, which involves integrating cognitive psychotherapy within spiritual framework. Here, beyond familial support various spiritual and religious leaders and institutions play a pivotal role in providing essential assistance for individuals seeking help to cope with the challenges of stressful life. These resources contribute to instilling a sense of belongingness and purpose, guiding individuals towards more profound and meaningful life objectives. India has made substantial contributions to the field of psychotherapy, particularly in the introduction of third-wave therapies like mindfulness-based therapies. It is worth noting that mindfulness techniques, frequently integrated with conventional cognitive behavioral therapy, trace their lineage to the ancient practice of meditation, which aims to achieve a balance and coordination of mind, body and consciousness *(Bhargava et al., 2017)*.

To adapt psychotherapy in Indian context, it is crucial to integrate cultural sensitivity and address these barriers. Tailoring psychoeducation programs to enhance awareness about mental health emphasizing its biological basis, could help combat misconceptions. Education campaigns emphasizing the effectiveness of psychotherapy. Collaborating with religious and spiritual leaders to reduce stigma and encourage seeking professional help may be effective *(Mendenhall et al., 2014)*. Additionally, incorporating family members in the therapeutic process and integrating traditional healing practices within a therapeutic framework could enhance acceptance. Providing affordable options such as community based, or online therapy can make it more accessible. Additionally, tailoring therapeutic approaches to align with cultural norms and emphasizing shorter, focused interventions may address the preference for quicker relief.

PSYCHOTHERAPY TRAINING AND PRACTICE IN INDIA

The WHO report from 2017 underscores a concerning gap between the low rate of psychologists (0.07 per 100,000) and the limited training opportunities (0.010 per 100,000) in India *(Mental Health Atlas 2017 Country Profile)*. This discrepancy is particularly significant given the higher prevalence of mental health illnesses per 100,000 in comparison to many other countries. Addressing this imbalance is crucial for enhancing mental health care and support in the country. The limited number of psychologists in India, coupled with the higher prevalence of mental health issues has led to an increased focus on training opportunities in psychotherapeutic approaches. While master's level training in clinical and counseling psychology includes modules on various psychotherapies, postgraduate diplomas and certificate courses also offer specialized skill-based learning. However, the courses are noted to be inadequate and theoretical, often lacking sufficient supervision. This highlights a need for more comprehensive and practical training to address the growing mental health challenges in the country *(Kalra, 2020)*. The psychotherapy training requires adequate supervision. But the absence of proper supervision is often acknowledged in India and results in therapists lacking essential skills. The importance of active, supervised training in psychotherapy for junior and trainee psychiatrists, highlighting the need for a more structured approach should be emphasized.

Supervision becomes even more challenging in India due to the multilingual nature of patients, trainees, and trainers. The group supervision is feasible and acceptable in a general hospital psychiatry setup in India, although it is acknowledged that group supervision cannot fully replace individual supervision. The call for improved and structured supervision underscores the ongoing efforts to enhance the quality of psychotherapy training in the country *(Manickam, et al., 2010)*.

The training landscape for psychotherapists in India involves specialized programs, such as the 1 year full-time clinical fellowship in CBT at National Institute of Mental Health and Neurosciences Hospital (NIMHANS), specifically designed for postgraduates with an MPhil in Clinical Psychology. However, the availability of seats is limited, with only four currently offered. Psychotherapy training in India is limited to cognitive behavior therapy and rational emotive behavior therapy. Therapies that are more deeply rooted like psychoanalytic psychotherapy has received minimum attention.

For psychiatry postgraduates, training in psychotherapy is constrained by factors like a predominant emphasis on pharmacological management, time constraints, and a lack of supervised trainers. Recognition of the importance of psychotherapy is widespread among mental health professionals in India. Some postgraduate programs in training institutes acknowledge this significance by incorporating relevant psychotherapeutic skills into their curriculum. The inclusion of supervised therapy as an essential component of training reflects a commitment to providing more holistic and effective treatment for patients. While recognizing the importance of psychotherapy, its incorporation into the psychiatry curriculum is limited *(Rao, 1985)*.

Psychologists in India often lean towards an eclectic approach, combining various therapeutic modalities to address diverse problems, rather than specializing in a single approach *(Kumar & Gupta, 2012)*. While CBT holds a central role in training, its popularity and success have made it a cornerstone in addressing various mental disorders. Its prevalence extends across different settings, from private practice, counseling and therapy centers, clinics, nonprofit organizations, schools, colleges to corporate organizations, showcasing its adaptability. The proliferation of CBT-driven counseling centers in urban areas highlights the demand for structured therapeutic approaches. Corporate recognition of work-life balance further emphasizes the integration of CBT with industrial/organizational psychologists applying its principles. However, the scenario is distinct in rural areas, where reliance on government hospitals and nonprofit organizations often facilitated by social worker, remains the primary avenue for mental health services. This dual landscape suggests a need for tailored strategies—reinforcing CBT training in urban settings and enhancing access to diverse therapeutic modalities in rural areas fostering a comprehensive and inclusive mental health support system across the country.

NATIONAL MEDICAL COMMISSION GUIDELINES AND PSYCHOTHERAPY TRAINING

National Medical Commission (NMC) Postgraduate Medical Education Board released new guidelines for the curriculum of different subjects on 5th August, 2022. Guidelines for competency-based postgraduate training program for MD in Psychiatry mentioned training in psychotherapy at few places in the curriculum.

The first mention of psychotherapy involves that the psychiatry trainee should be able to perform following psychotherapy under supervision: (1) Behavior therapy, (2) Family therapy, (3) Interpersonal therapy, (4) Cognitive behavior therapy and other newer therapies, (5) First level psychological intervention for sexual abuse, sexual assault, and domestic violence, and (6) Genetic counseling. The guidelines also mention about incorporation of small group tutorials supervised by a consultant for case presentation and discussion adds a practical dimension to the training. This approach can facilitate a comprehensive understanding of psychotherapy management.

It appears that the guidelines for the Competency-based Postgraduate Training Program for MD in Psychiatry emphasize a diverse range of psychotherapies without specifying minimum case requirements or supervision details. The absence of guidelines on the number of therapy hours and the supervisor's qualifications may leave room for interpretation. Additionally, the lack of practical demonstration in the examination format raises questions about the assessment of psychotherapy skills. It might be beneficial to seek clarification or additional information from the relevant authorities to ensure a comprehensive understanding of the expectations for psychotherapy training in MD (Psychiatry) (*Guidelines for Competency-based Postgraduate Training Program for MD in Psychiatry*, 2021).

PSYCHOTHERAPY COURSES IN INDIA

The training landscape in India for cognitive-behavioral therapies (CBT and REBT) includes informal certificate or diploma courses offered by some organizations. It is important to note that these courses are not affiliated or recognized by the parent institutes, namely the Beck Institute for Cognitive Behavior Therapy or Albert Ellis Institute (AEI) in the USA. The Indian Association for CBT *(Indian Association of Cognitive Behaviour Therapy,* n.d.*)*, and the CARE Institute of Behavioural Sciences in Chennai, Tamil Nadu are some other institutes which provide relevant training in psychotherapeutic skills, acknowledging the holistic benefits for patient treatment. Certain mental health centers provide more structured training in CBT, often conducted by trainers certified abroad and mentored by them from the parent institutes. The scarcity of skill-based training and supervision in psychotherapy is noted to impact the credibility of professionals in India *(Kumar & Gupta, 2012)*. Additionally, study in 2019 revealed that the quality of formal CBT training workshops, along with supervision and an increased number of trained professionals, influenced the number of consultations in a teaching hospital in Northern India *(Gupta et al., 2019)*.

The current scenario for clinical psychologists, counselors, and other mental health professionals in India is characterized by a lack of regulatory structure. There is no licensing system, central professional agency, or legal/governmental branch to enforce regulations. This absence of oversight extends to the practice, training, and competence of mental health professionals, contributing to a complex and unregulated landscape in the field of psychotherapy *(Kumar & Gupta, 2012)*.

In India, the absence of nationally standardized ethical guidelines for psychotherapists has led to efforts at organizational and regional levels to establish professional regulations. The Indian Association of Clinical Psychologists (IACP) is one such independent organization working toward this goal. The IACP has taken a step by formulating professional ethics based on the principles of the American Psychological Association (APA) for its members, as outlined in studies by Sathyanarayanan, 2018 and Misra & Rizvi, 2012. While these initiatives represent progress, comprehensive national standards are yet to be established in the field.

The Mental Healthcare Act of 2017 in India, a revision of the previous Mental Healthcare Bill, emphasizes the rights of the mentally ill and is aligned with the WHO's Rights of Persons with Disabilities (UNCRPD) *(Mishra & Galhotra, 2018)*. However, the guidelines in the Mental Healthcare Act (MHA) primarily focus on pharmacotherapy and hospitalization. Notably, the Act lacks specific clauses addressing psychotherapy and lacks regulations for mental health professionals other than psychiatrists. The only provision mentioning psychological services stipulates who is a clinical psychologist, he/she must hold a postgraduate degree in clinical psychology and be a member of the Rehabilitation Council of India (RCI) [*Mental Health Care Act 2017 Chapter 1, section 2 (g) p. 2*].

The RCI is expected to regulate the practices of professionals treating patients with physical and psychological disabilities, including mental illnesses once the MHA comes into practice in respective states. Originally established as a regulatory body for professionals working with differently abled individuals, the RCI now extends its code of ethics to include clinical psychologists in the country. The Rehabilitation Council of India Act of 1993 serves as the legal framework, prohibiting certain practices to ensure ethical standards in the field.

LACK OF REGULATIONS FOR PSYCHOTHERAPY PRACTICE IN INDIA

The lack of regulations for psychotherapy in India stems from several factors, including:

- *Priority to pharmacotherapy:* The predominant emphasis on pharmacotherapy as the primary or sole treatment for psychiatric disorders has contributed to the absence of specific regulations for psychotherapy.
- *Lack of consensus:* There is a lack of consensus among professionals regarding the definition of psychotherapy and who qualifies as a psychotherapist or counselor. Questions arise about the distinctions between counseling and psychotherapy, and a clear legal definition is lacking.
- *Cultural debate:* Debates persist about the applicability of "Western" therapies in Indian culture, adding to confusion about the qualifications of a psychotherapist.
- *Resistance to norms:* Some professionals may resist establishing norms due to discomfort with additional procedures, concerns about restrictions on practices, anxiety about ethical issues, and a lack of trust in other professionals to establish fair norms.
- *Focus on awareness:* Psychotherapists have prioritized creating awareness about psychotherapy in the general population rather than establishing a universally approved professional agency with legal enforcement power.
- *Need for accountability:* There is a recognized need for a mechanism to hold psychologists accountable nationwide, with a formal code of conduct specifying behavioral standards.

Despite the recognition and efforts by experienced professionals to promote a uniform code of conduct and a central regulatory agency, these endeavors have fallen short. The establishment of a professional body for standardization, enforcement, and guidance in resolving ethical issues is deemed essential to address the current gaps in psychotherapy regulations in India.

CHALLENGES IN THE REALM OF PSYCHOTHERAPY TRAINING IN INDIA

- *Subjectivity and individualism:* Psychotherapy is inherently subjective and individualistic, making it a complex skill to impart uniformly.
- *Extended training time:* The challenge of limited time for effective psychotherapy training, exacerbated by high patient loads in Indian hospitals, is indeed a significant concern. Balancing the demands of patient care with comprehensive training needs poses a practical challenge. There is also a lack of specialized training in child and adolescent psychotherapy, which needs special expertise and techniques. It might be worthwhile to advocate for resource allocation and restructuring training programs to accommodate the essential aspects of psychotherapy. Addressing these systemic issues could contribute to better integration of psychotherapy training into postgraduate programs, ultimately bridging the gap between the demand for psychological intervention and the availability of trained professionals.
- *Lack of inclination:* Not all trainees may have a natural inclination or interest in pursuing psychotherapy as part of their professional development.
- *Availability of committed trainers:* The limited availability of trainers committed to psychotherapeutic skills and the lack of consensus on whether psychiatrists or psychologists should supervise training pose significant challenges. This is compounded by the fact that many psychiatrists may not have received formal training in psychotherapy themselves. Addressing these issues may require advocacy for increased training opportunities, collaboration between psychiatrists and psychologists, and possibly, the development of specific training programs for psychiatrists in psychotherapy. Advocating for clearer guidelines on supervision qualifications could also contribute to a more effective training environment.
- *Few training centers:* The limited number of recognized training centers, coupled with a focus primarily only on cognitive behavior therapy, underscores a significant gap in the availability of diverse and comprehensive psychotherapy training opportunities. Advocacy for the accreditation of more training centers and diversification of therapeutic approaches could enhance access to quality training. Collaborative efforts between relevant authorities and mental health professionals might help

address these limitations, ensuring a broader range of psychotherapeutic skills are cultivated among trainees.

- *Impracticability of analysis:* Some psychoanalytically-oriented approaches may require impractical levels of analysis of the trainee, making certain methods challenging to implement.
- *Novelty of concepts:* Trainees may encounter novel psychological and philosophical concepts, adding a layer of complexity to the learning process.
- *Eclectic approach:* The prevalence of eclectic approaches in psychotherapy does present challenges in developing standardized training modules, as practitioners draw from diverse methods. Crafting a universally applicable curriculum becomes intricate when considering the varied techniques employed by therapists in their eclectic practices. The prevalence of eclectic approaches in psychotherapy does present challenges in developing standardized training modules, as practitioners draw from diverse methods. Crafting a universally applicable curriculum becomes intricate when considering the varied techniques employed by therapists in their eclectic practices. The integration of diverse therapeutic techniques and alternative therapies can complicate efforts to conduct rigorous evidence-based studies. The field's eclecticism poses challenges in standardizing interventions for research, potentially impacting the establishment of clear cause-and-effect relationships.
- *Absence of regulation and monitoring of psychotherapy training:* The absence of a structured mechanism for monitoring, evaluating, and accrediting training programs in psychotherapy poses challenges. Additionally, the lack of provisions for legislation and insurance for practitioners further complicates the field. While existing training courses may deepen knowledge, they often fall short in effectively enhancing skill literacy among trainees.

These challenges collectively underscore the need for concerted efforts to address training gaps, enhance resources, and foster a more supportive environment for psychotherapy education in the country *(Manickam et al., 2010) (Kishore et al., 2010)*.

RESEARCH ON PSYCHOTHERAPY IN INDIA

The research in psychotherapy is very limited in India. Most of the research is conducted on cognitive behavior therapy and rational emotive behavior therapy *(Manickam 2010 et al., 2010)*. The research in India is mainly limited to case studies and case series. The current research landscape in psychotherapy reveals notable trends. Studies often center around clinical populations or those with physical ailments, potentially due to easier access or a crisis intervention focus over prevention. Methodologically, the emphasis is on overall therapy efficacy with limited exploration of specific therapy components. Evaluations primarily target therapy outcomes rather than the therapeutic process itself (*Kuruvilla, 2010*). Bridging this gap could enhance understanding and application. Furthermore, exploring the cross-cultural application of therapies like REBT in India can contribute to a more comprehensive perspective, given the current low acceptance despite its global evidence-based status (*Cognitive Behavioral Therapy in a Global Context | Springer Link*, n.d.).

The scarcity of psychotherapeutic literature can be attributed to several factors, including a shortage of training centers, inadequate research instruments, time constraints, facility limitations, and insufficient supervised training. Additionally, client perspectives on confidentiality, privacy, and stigma may also contribute to a reluctance to participate in research studies, further limiting the available literature in the field of psychotherapy.

Encouraging postgraduate students to delve into psychotherapy research, including single case studies and treatment-based studies, is crucial for advancing evidence-based practices. Establishing journals in India that focus exclusively on psychotherapeutic interventions could provide a platform for researchers to share insights and contribute to the development of culturally sensitive approaches. This could foster a richer understanding of mental health and enhance the relevance of psychotherapy in the Indian context (*Lodha & De Sousa, 2020*).

CHALLENGES IN THE DELIVERY OF EVIDENCE-BASED PSYCHOLOGICAL THERAPIES IN INDIA

***Challenge 1:* The acceptance of psychotherapy as a valid psychiatric treatment In India—there has been a prevalent belief that doctors primarily prescribe medications to treat psychiatric disorders**

Consequently, there is a widespread reluctance to accept psychotherapy as a legitimate form of psychiatric treatment. Many patients seeking psychiatric care typically expect to receive medication and brief advice from their doctor, with little inclination to engage in conversations to explore and understand the underlying factors contributing to their issues. This reluctance is fueled by various factors including time and financial constraints, hesitancy to open to a doctor, and the misconception that counseling and psychotherapy alone are insufficient for healing. As a result, there is a lack of trust among patients in the effectiveness of psychotherapy as a treatment option. Some argue that mere words will not propel us forward, advocating for medications and injections as tangible solutions over the contemplative exercise of validating one's thoughts in therapy. Many seeking psychiatric aid are family providers, pressed for time and deterred by the commitment of regular sessions. To surmount this, psychiatrists ingeniously embed 15–20 minute "mini-sessions" within consultations, subtly weaving diverse psychotherapeutic perspectives and techniques.

***Challenge 2:* Mismatch between demand and need for psychotherapy**
The 2015–2016 National Mental Health Survey (NMHS) revealed a lifetime-weighted prevalence of 13.7% for mental morbidity in India, with an average of 10.6% at the time. The survey identified a substantial treatment gap, ranging from 70 to 92% for various disorders. Notably, common mental disorders had an 85% treatment gap, severe mental disorders a 73.6% gap, and psychosis a 75.5% gap, among others.

These findings imply a substantial demand for psychiatric services and achieving comprehensive coverage under the National Mental Health Program (NMHP) across all districts in India may prove challenging. Moreover, there has been a rise in the crude prevalence and disability-adjusted life-years (DALYs) rate for depressive disorders, anxiety disorders, bipolar disorders, and schizophrenia in India from 1990 to 2017. During the same period, the proportional contribution of mental disorders to the overall disease burden in India has doubled.

Given the significant burden of mental disorders and the substantial treatment gap in pharmacological interventions, incorporating psychotherapy as a treatment modality seems challenging. The scarcity of trained personnel is particularly evident at the primary and secondary levels, making widespread delivery of therapy difficult. Even at the tertiary level, therapy is primarily accessible in a few government hospitals, further constrained by a limited number of psychologists.

***Challenge 3:* Explaining to patients how psychotherapy works and their ability to comprehend and understand the same**
The lack of a clear neurobiological mechanism and quantifiable markers for its effectiveness, the subjective nature of psychological change and the absence of tangible, measurable outcomes can indeed make it challenging for some patients to fully grasp and accept this therapeutic process. It is a complex interplay of cognitive, emotional, and behavioral factors, making psychotherapy more nuanced compared to the relatively straightforward mechanisms often associated with medication. Despite these challenges, many individuals benefit from the holistic approach that psychotherapy offers, emphasizing the importance of the therapeutic alliance and the exploration of thoughts and emotions.

***Challenge 4:* Limited emphasis on integrating psychotherapy into psychiatric practice**
Psychotherapy has not been integrated in the treatment process due to limited training emphasis, time constraints, and the influence of practice settings. The prioritization of biological approaches in training, coupled with

the demands of busy clinical environments, may contribute to psychiatrists leaning towards medication-based interventions. The scarcity of supervised psychotherapy practice during training and the practical limitations in private practice further impede the active incorporation of psychotherapy into psychiatrists' routines. It underscores the need for a more comprehensive and supportive framework to encourage psychiatrists to develop and maintain proficiency in psychotherapeutic skills, recognizing the value it brings to holistic patient care.

***Challenge 5:* The individualization of psychotherapy**
This emphasizes on the need for psychiatrists to adapt their approach based on individual patient dynamics. The varied communication styles, levels of engagement, and preferences among patients necessitate a flexible and personalized therapeutic strategy. The challenge lies in navigating this diversity, being attuned to each patient's unique needs, and adjusting the therapeutic style accordingly. It underscores the importance of honing a range of skills to effectively connect with different individuals and tailor psychotherapy to suit their personalities and therapeutic requirements.

***Challenge 6:* Choosing a school of psychotherapy and the perils of eclecticism**
The challenge of choosing the most suitable psychotherapeutic approach is indeed complex, particularly in diverse cultural settings like India. Specializing in a particular school of therapy provides a structured framework, but the eclectic approach recognizes the importance of tailoring interventions to individual needs. While eclecticism can offer flexibility, it may pose challenges in terms of patient expectations and perceptions. Striking a balance between a structured session-by-session model and adapting to the unique aspects of each patient's psychological makeup is crucial. This nuanced approach requires ongoing assessment and adjustment, considering both the psychiatrist's expertise and the patient's preferences for a more effective therapeutic alliance.

***Challenge 7:* Documentation and maintaining notes of therapy sessions**
Maintaining detailed documentation in psychotherapy is crucial, serving both as a record of progress and a legal safeguard. The challenge arises from time constraints and the potential difficulty in recalling specific details of past sessions, especially when patients seek records after an extended period. Establishing a systematic approach to documentation is essential, helping psychiatrists track the trajectory of therapy and ensuring a comprehensive record that can be referenced when needed. This not only supports transparency but also aids in providing a thorough account of the therapeutic journey in case of future inquiries or legal requirements.

***Challenge 8:* How to choose the right patient for psychotherapy**

Selecting the right patients for psychotherapy is indeed a delicate balance, and the success of therapy often hinges on the patient's mindset, willingness to engage, and level of psychological insight. The challenge lies in identifying those who possess the necessary qualities for effective engagement in psychotherapeutic processes. Limited training in this aspect adds to the complexity, emphasizing the need for a more structured approach to patient selection. Making the right choices can significantly impact both the patient's and therapist's confidence, contributing to positive outcomes and the efficient use of resources in private practice psychotherapy.

***Challenge 9:* The emergence of online psychotherapy**

The advent of online psychotherapy indeed expands access to mental health care, especially in developing regions. However, the lack of formal training, guidelines and a consensus on ethical and legal aspects poses challenges. Careful consideration of the moral and ethical dilemmas, along with awareness of the potential limitations of online platforms, is crucial for psychiatrists venturing into this realm. While online psychotherapy offers convenience, the absence of in-person interactions may limit personal observations. Balancing the benefits and challenges, especially when patients demand or are referred for pure online psychotherapy, requires a thoughtful and informed approach in office-based therapy settings. *(Lodha & De Sousa, 2018), (Bhola & Raguram, 2016).*

CONCLUSION

Psychotherapy has been a part of Indian culture from time immemorial in the form of spiritual and religious teachings. Providing mental health services to the large population of India has been a challenging task for mental health planners thus limiting the required focus on treatment modalities like psychotherapy. Further, challenges like the scarcity of trained professionals, limited training opportunities, and a preference for quick relief through pharmacological treatment also contribute to non-mainstream status of psychotherapy in addressing psychological disturbances. Currently research on psychotherapy in India also remains limited. Addressing these challenges is crucial for enhancing the recognition and accessibility of psychotherapy in the country.

FURTHER READING

1. Bhargava R, Kumar N, Gupta A. Indian perspective on psychotherapy: cultural issues. J Contemp Psychother. 2017;47:95-103. [online] Available from https://doi.org/10.1007/s10879-016-9348-1 [Last accessed December, 2023].
2. Bhatia SC, Madabushi J, Kolli V, Bhatia SK, Madaan V. The Bhagavad Gita and contemporary psychotherapies. Indian J Psychiatry. 2013;55(Suppl 2):

S315-S321. [online] Available from https://doi.org/10.4103/0019-5545.105557 [Last accessed December, 2023].

3. Bhola P, Raguram A (Eds). Ethical Issues in Counselling and Psychotherapy Practice. Springer; 2016. [online] Available from https://doi.org/10.1007/978-981-10-1808-4 [Last accessed December, 2023].
4. Guidelines for Competency-based Postgraduate Training Programme for MD in Psychiatry. NMC; 2021.
5. Gupta AK, Sharma E, Kar SK, Tripathi A, Reeves T, Arjundas R, et al. (2019). Training and Clinical Impact of Cognitive Behaviour Therapy Workshops in a Teaching Hospital in North India. Indian J Psychol Med. 2019;41(4):343-7. [online] Available from https://doi.org/10.4103/IJPSYM.IJPSYM_183_18 [Last accessed December, 2023].
6. IACBT. (n.d.). Retrieved 1 November 2023. [online] Available from https://www.iacbt.org/about-us.html [Last accessed December, 2023].
7. Kalra V (n.d.). Psychotherapy Model for the Training of Counselors in India.
8. Kishore ANR., Shaji KS, Praveenlal K. Revalidation: Are we Meeting Training Needs? Training and its Influence on the Practice of Child Psychiatry and Psychotherapy. Indian J Psychol Med. 2010;32(1):3-6. [online] Available from https://doi.org/10.4103/0253-7176.70515 [Last accessed December, 2023].
9. Kumar N, Gupta P. Cognitive Behaviour Therapy in India: Adaptations, Beliefs and Challenges. In: Naeem F, Kingdon D (Eds). Cognitive Behaviour Therapy in Non-Western Cultures. Nova Science Publishers Inc. New York, USA; 2012. pp. 61-77.
10. Kuruvilla K. Indian contribution to behavior therapy. Indian J Psychiatry. 2010;52(Suppl 1):S371. [online] Available from https://doi.org/10.4103/0019-5545.69271 [Last accessed December, 2023].
11. Lodha P, De Sousa A. Challenges for Office Psychotherapy Practice in India. Annals of Indian Psychiatry. 2018;2(1):6. [online] Available from https://doi.org/10.4103/aip.aip_6_18 [Last accessed December, 2023].
12. Lodha P, De Sousa A. Psychotherapy research in India: A distant dream. Indian J Psychiatry. 2022;62(1):106-7. [online] Available from https://doi.org/10.4103/psychiatry. Indian J Psychiatry_240_19 [Last accessed December, 2023].
13. Manickam LSS. Psychotherapy in India Indian J Psychiatry. 2010;52(Suppl 1):S366-S370. [online] Available from https://www.ncbi.nlm.nih.gov/pmc/articles/PMC3146194/[Last accessed December, 2023].
14. Mendenhall E, De Silva MJ, Hanlon C, Petersen I, Shidhaye R, Jordans M, et al. Acceptability and feasibility of using non-specialist health workers to deliver mental health care: Stakeholder perceptions from the PRIME district sites in Ethiopia, India, Nepal, South Africa, and Uganda. Social Science & Medicine. 2014;118:33-42. [online] Available from https://doi.org/10.1016/j.socscimed.2014.07.057 [Last accessed December, 2023].
15. Mental Health Atlas 2017 Country Profile: India. Retrieved 28 November 2023. [online] Available from https://www.who.int/publications/m/item/mental-health-atlas-2017-country-profile-india [Last accessed December, 2023].
16. Mental Health Care Act 2017. [online] Available from https://www.indiacode.nic.in/bitstream/123456789/2249/1/A2017-10.pdf [Last accessed December, 2023].

17. Mishra A, Galhotra A. Mental Healthcare Act 2017: Need to Wait and Watch. Int J App Basic Med Res. 2018;8(2):67. [online] Available from https://doi.org/10.4103/ijabmr.IJABMR_328_17 [Last accessed December, 2023].
18. Misra RK, Rizvi SH. Clinical Psychology in India: A Meta-analytic Review. Int J Psychol Stud. 2012;4(4):18. [online] Available from https://doi.org/10.5539/ijps.v4n4p18 [Last accessed December, 2023].
19. Neki JS. Psychotherapy in India: Past, Present, and Future. Am J Psychother. 1975;29(1):92-100. [online] Available from https://doi.org/10.1176/appi.psychotherapy.1975.29.1.92 [Last accessed December, 2023].
20. Rao AV. Psychotherapy in the Indian Context. In: P Pichot, P Berner, R Wolf, K Thau (Eds). Psychiatry the State of the Art, Volume 4, Springer US. Psychother and Psychosom Med. 1985;141-6. [online] Available from https://doi.org/10.1007/978-1-4684-4697-5_25 [Last accessed December, 2023].
21. Sathyanarayanan V. Ethics in psychotherapy and counselling practice: The Indian scenario. Indian J Med Ethics; 2018. [online] Available from https://doi.org/10.20529/IJME.2018.013 [Last accessed December, 2023].
22. Terjesen MD, Doyle KA. Cognitive Behavioral Therapy in a Global Context. Springer Link. (n.d.); 2023. [online] Available from https://link.springer.com/book/10.1007/978-3-030-82555-3 [Last accessed December, 2023].
23. The burden of mental disorders across the states of India: The Global Burden of Disease Study 1990–2017. (2020). Lancet Psychiatr. 2020;7(2):148-61. [online] Available from: https://doi.org/10.1016/S2215-0366(19)30475-4 [Last accessed December, 2023].
24. Union Budget for Mental Health 2023-2024. (n.d.). [online] Available from https://cmhlp.org/wp-content/uploads/2023/02/Budget-Brief-2023-v3.pdf [Last accessed December, 2023].
25. World Mental Health Report 2022. [online] Available from https://iris.who.int/bitstream/handle/10665/356119/9789240049338-eng.pdf?sequence=1 [Last accessed December, 2023].

4

CHAPTER

Psychotherapy in Underprivileged Persons from Low Socioeconomic Status and Illiteracy

Advait Dixit, Krishna Prasad Muliyala, Geetha Desai

ABSTRACT

Psychotherapy is an effective tool in the treatment of various mental illnesses (MI). Psychotherapy in the context of poverty and low literacy presents distinctive challenges. Poverty and illiteracy share a complex and bidirectional relationship with MI. The socioeconomic struggles of low-income populations introduce practical barriers, such as the costs of psychotherapy, transportation costs and the inherent challenge of adhering to therapy amidst unpredictable work schedules. Concurrently, stigma surrounding mental health often necessitates primary care rather than specialized mental health care. Psychotherapy historically caters to more privileged classes and exemplifies existing inequities in mental health care. Global disparities in mental health workforce distribution hinder accessibility, particularly in low-and middle-income countries. Despite these challenges, an emerging body of evidence points towards the efficacy of psychotherapy in addressing the mental health needs of low-income. There is a need for tailored interventions, heightened mental health literacy, and innovative strategies to address the multifaceted challenges encountered by illiterate and people with low-income status.

Keywords: Psychotherapy, Underprivileged, Low socioeconomic status, Illiteracy

INTRODUCTION

Socioeconomically disadvantaged people constitute a large and growing proportion of people in low- and middle-income countries (LMICs); between 2.5% of the population and 29.5% of people live in poverty based on different estimates in India, an LMIC. Data from India's 2011 census shows that about 269 million people live in poverty, which makes up 22% of the population.[1] Illiteracy, on the other hand, is a complex and multifaceted issue. According to the Indian census data, the literacy rate for men stood at 82.4%, and the literacy rate for women stood at 65.8%. About 25% of the population in India is illiterate.[2]

Low income and poverty are known risk factors for mental illnesses. Exposure to poverty contributes significantly to the onset of major depression. The link between young age, interpersonal violence, low-income status, and the development of post-traumatic stress disorder (PTSD) is well established.[3,4] A large population-based study analyzed the association of common mental disorders (CMDs) with different sociodemographic determinants in a representative sample of about 5700 Indian women wherein, they found a positive between lower educational status, a lower standard of living, alcohol use in the spouse, intimate partner violence with CMDs.[5] Poverty and MI share a bidirectional association. Even after accounting for other factors, there are pointers to the connection between adverse economic events and severe mental illnesses (SMIs), depression, PTSD, and anxiety disorders.[6-8]

The social causation hypothesis suggests that poverty increases the chances of MI due to increased stress, lack of opportunity, social exclusion, poor support systems and high incidence of trauma and violence. On the other hand, the social selection or social drift theory postulates that persons with MI have higher odds of moving into or staying in poverty due to higher healthcare costs, lower productivity, stigma, the inability to find work and the loss of income. While the social selection theory may be more relevant to conditions like schizophrenia and intellectual disability, the social causation pathway may be more appropriate to CMDs.

Numerous evidence-based psychosocial treatments exist for MI, and specific psychotherapies in recent times have been recommended as stand-alone treatments or as adjuncts to pharmacotherapy. There are significant differences between populations with greater resources and those who are from the lower-income group in terms of the accessibility, utilization, and availability of psychotherapy services.

SOCIOECONOMIC STATUS AND PSYCHOPATHOLOGY

Common mental disorders like depression, anxiety, and substance use disorders have been associated with social position. Educational attainment and mathematical ability are protective factors for psychiatric disorders. A study by Wadsworth and Achenbach (2005) tested two mechanisms of how low socioeconomic status (SES) may cause psychopathology in children and youth. The study found that low SES was associated with an increased risk of developing clinical elevations on several psychological syndromes, such as anxiety/depression, somatic complaints, thought problems, and delinquent and aggressive suggesting that low SES exposes children and youth to more stressors and adversities that trigger psychological problems. The study also found that low SES was associated with less improvement in some psychological syndromes, such as being withdrawn and somatic complaints, suggesting that low SES limits access to resources and opportunities that facilitate recovery from psychological problems.[9] The social causation of psychopathology states the need for interventions tailored to the unique problems caused and perpetuated by the individual's socioeconomic status. Somatization (psychological conflict transformed into bodily symptoms) and somatization tendency (proclivity to report somatic symptoms) have been associated with poverty in both high and low-middle-income countries.[10] Dissociative disorders do correlate with lower socioeconomic status and low educational attainment.[11,12] Genetic findings related to psychopathology and psychosocial factors may be mediated by genetic overlap with literacy and socioeconomic status.[13]

ACCESS TO MENTAL HEALTH CARE AND PSYCHOLOGICAL METHODS OF TREATMENT

Despite their need, many low-income individuals do not receive mental healthcare. Only 13% of low-income people who were likely to have experienced trauma had received therapy linked to trauma, even though 22% of them fulfilled the criteria for PTSD.[14] Less service utilization is associated with other characteristics such as social isolation, neighborhood deprivation, and single-parent status.[15]

Higher incomes, employment status, and educational attainment were all linked to more frequent usage of private psychotherapy when the client paid 40–100 GBP per session. Even though public psychotherapy was less accessible due to referral requirements and longer wait times for treatment, individuals with lower incomes, educational levels, and professional status utilized it more frequently.[16] In France, a study looked at how life events, mental health, and sociodemographic traits—like education—affect the use of psychotherapy. Most of the study participants were middle-class, working individuals having health insurance. The use of psychotherapy in varying degrees of psychiatric problems was positively correlated with education, even though the research population had high-quality insurance coverage and was well-informed about the existing systems.[17] The German statutory health insurance registration data analysis showed that outpatient psychotherapy treatment was significantly under-covered in lower socioeconomic groups. The qualification of an individual positively correlated with psychotherapy utilization rates. The study's key finding is that psychotherapists should focus more on their clients from lower socioeconomic backgrounds and modify their treatments for those with less language fluency. Enhancing mental health literacy at the community level will help reduce barriers to psychotherapy and consequently increase its use.[18] Evidence of income-based disparities in the use of psychotherapy has also been found in Australia and Canada.[19] Despite the differences in the delivery systems, there was a greater unmet need for psychotherapy in low-income groups in both nations. While Australia has offered universally accessible psychotherapy since the Better Access reform in 2006, Canada maintains a two-tier system that drives up the expense of psychotherapy for those with low incomes. The findings showed that despite the change, there were also income-based disparities in psychotherapy in Australia.[19]

A study by Hines-Martin et al. (2003) categorized barriers to mental healthcare at three levels—Individual, Environmental, and Institutional. Individual barriers reflected things that kept people from asking for assistance when they needed it. Environmental barriers represented things in the affected people's surroundings that hindered or made it harder to ask for assistance. Institutional barriers were those that prevented the participants from getting the resources that they had identified. The findings from the study concluded that individual barriers (beliefs, financial obstacles, knowledge about the illness) were the most significant in preventing access to mental health services.[20]

BARRIERS TO ACCESSING PSYCHOTHERAPY

The basic needs of the people from low-income bracket are unmet. Hence, there is often a debate about whether the therapist should focus on concepts like self-reflection, self-esteem, and self-actualization. If we allude to Maslow's theory of motivation, self-actualization is at the top of the pyramid, with food safety at the bottom. It gives a false impression that low-income individuals might not be suitable for psychotherapy, where the goal is to address self-esteem and self-actualization. This approach is paternalistic as the therapists are deciding the needs of these individuals.[21]

Some practical barriers the patients are face lack of public transportation or expensive transportation and missed daily wages. Getting help could feel overwhelming, especially since it takes time, which they do not always have. Therapists usually expect their clients to attend frequent sessions at a clinic or office. Still, if the patients are working, they can have shift work with unpredictable schedules that prevent them from committing to a specific time and location each week. People with low incomes usually have no choice but to use public transport, which can be expensive and often unpredictable regarding timings and arrivals. The expense and distance of travel for appointments may prevent people with low incomes in rural areas from attending regular therapy sessions. Weekly therapy sessions take a significant toll on the time and finances of people with low income.

Low-income patients are more likely to attend primary care physicians than specialized mental health care settings due to stigma. However, primary care physicians lack training in psychotherapy, and the consultation time is less. They are unlikely to have enough time to identify and treat mental health issues, particularly in overcrowded settings where people with limited resources obtain healthcare. Primary care providers may be reluctant to inquire too deeply into emotional issues. Many are also concerned that, should they detect mental health issues in patients, they may not know to whom to report them.[22] In addition to the challenges brought on by poverty, the additional burden of psychiatric disorders may reduce help-seeking. However, there is conflicting data about the importance of stigma as a therapeutic barrier for the impoverished. Although quantitative survey and interview data frequently paint a different picture, much qualitative research documents significant stigma among persons who belong to the low-income bracket.[23,24]

Psychoanalysis and Social Class

Rory du Plessis has offered interesting perspectives on social class and psychoanalysis. Psychotherapy has historically and theoretically neglected and dismissed the low-income individuals as unsuitable candidates for treatment. Since its inception, psychotherapy has been a privilege catering to the middle and higher classes. Even the works of pioneers of psychoanalysis like Freud and Jung have primarily involved the privileged classes. There is an "inherent attitudinal bias amongst psychotherapists where the low-income individuals are viewed to have deficits in their *psychic life*, lacking desires and intellectual capabilities" and thus are deemed unfit for psychotherapeutic interventions. It is in stark contrast with the increasing body of evidence that points towards the effectiveness of psychotherapy in low-income individuals.[25]

UNDERSTANDING THE DISADVANTAGED: A SOCIAL-ECOLOGICAL VIEW

Service providers frequently operate under the premise that a family will seek treatment if they genuinely want to improve. This presumption must consider the numerous problems, many families must face before receiving assistance. People living in poverty might need more access to telephones, Internet and transportation that come in the way of seeking appointments and services. The risk factors responsible for poverty in the family can be described at four levels: ontogenetic or individual, microsystem (family, home, school, or clinic settings), exosystem (community), and macrosystem (cultural). Ecological theorists understand risk factors within the individual and across social-ecological systems. A few examples of individual elements are age, gender, race, and the severity of the symptoms.

On the other hand, people are active participants in microsystems, which are immediate environment settings that affect people's behavior and wellbeing. The mesosystem, which depicts the degree of unity or overlap between different areas of an individual's environment, is linked to the microsystems. The exosystem, or community level, usually includes more general communal features that impact individual and family life, such as the accessibility of services for education and recreation.[15] Dropping out of school is common among low-income families, who are less likely to receive support. Poor outcomes from therapy are also associated with socioeconomic disadvantage.[26] Exosystem-level community factors can also hamper access to and use of services. For instance, it is common for rural communities to lack specialized resources and struggle to draw in qualified specialists. Rural families are more likely to experience insurance coverage issues, must travel farther to access services, and are more likely to be socially isolated, all of which raise the risk that they will not start treatment or fail to complete it. Poverty is linked with gender disparities, religious and ethnic minorities, substance use, conduct issues in childhood and domestic violence; the intersection of these factors is the structural driver of poverty and inequality. An intersectional approach can help us develop more inclusive policies that address the diverse needs of impoverished people to promote their empowerment.[27]

WORKING WITH LOW-INCOME CLIENTS

As reported in a qualitative study, therapists working with low-income clients have developed strategies for addressing power dynamics, managing boundaries, and addressing external stressors as part of the therapeutic process.[28] Therapists used empowerment and advocacy approaches to help their clients develop their voice and agency to address power dynamics. Therapists have adjusted boundaries to meet the client's needs and preferences rather than following rigid or standardized rules. Considering the context and culture of their clients and the potential benefits and risks of boundary crossings are other essential considerations in psychotherapy with people with low incomes.

Incorporating the assessment and intervention of external stressors, such as poverty, violence, discrimination, and oppression, into the therapeutic process can help clients access and navigate other resources and services that can address their basic and social needs. Having values-based commitment, experience, knowledge, empathy, self-awareness, and coping skills for working with this population is essential.[28]

RECOMMENDATIONS AND EVIDENCE-BASED APPROACH

The Evidence-based Approach to Overcoming Barriers

Evidence-based solutions for psychotherapists who want to work with this population involve:

- Understanding the diverse and unique needs of patients who are economically deprived, such as coping with trauma, stress, violence, discrimination and stigma. Communicating effectively with patients with different languages, cultures, values, and beliefs.
- They are dealing with payment-related issues, offering sliding scale or pro bono services, and setting up a policy for financial constraints.
- They are developing cultural competence, sensitivity, and ethical and professional standards when working with this population.

The psychotherapists who work with this population make a positive difference in the lives of their clients and communities and enrich their own personal and professional growth.

Saeromi Kim (2012) has emphasized the importance of assessing social class comprehensively and continuously using multiple and complex variables, such as income, education, occupation, assets, debt, social mobility, and subjective social status. Social class intersects with other sociocultural dimensions of identity, such as race, ethnicity, gender, age, and immigration status. Understanding clients' class status and identity, such as how they perceive and identify themselves with others, how they cope with class-related stressors, and how they view their opportunities and challenges, is important in psychotherapy. Some ways to manage the differences in social class between therapists and clients include practising critical self-reflection, openly acknowledging differences, and incorporating community approaches.[29]

Adapting psychotherapies to the needs of persons with mental health difficulties needs to focus on understanding the context. Different schools of psychotherapy have been considered for the same MI. Starting from psychoanalysis to the current third wave of cognitive behavioral therapies, the list has been endless. Across all forms of psychotherapies, common psychotherapeutic factors are pertinent for improving outcomes. Rigid principles of different schools of psychotherapy might be challenging to adapt to the needs of persons who are impoverished and illiterate.

Adaptations of briefer psychodynamic psychotherapies, IPT and CBT need to consider the context, culture, economic factors, literacy, and the availability of resources.[30,31]

Task-shifting to Address the Gap

To address the scarcity of resources of trained professionals, task-shifting, which "is a process of allocation of tasks from more specialized to less specialized healthcare workers wherever appropriate", has been considered. Some studies of the delivery of psychological intervention by Lay Healthcare Workers (LHWs) and peer-led programs have been shown to positively impact the reduction of overall costs, better retention of clients, and improvements in quality of life.[32] Early experiences with the Tuko Pamoja (we are together) intervention in Sub-Saharan Africa in training LHWs have demonstrated improvement in fidelity, acceptability, and clinical competencies in a pilot study.[33] Despite the enthusiasm surrounding task shifting to address the gap in mental health care in low-income people, robust studies looking at long-term effects and evidence of direct comparisons between the delivery of interventions by specialized professionals and LHWs are lacking. Teaching problem-solving techniques, behavioral activation, and supportive psychotherapy principles may be practical in resource-constrained settings and can be delivered by primary care physicians and lay counselors.

Indian Scenario

Since its inception, the National Mental Health Programme (NMHP) aimed to ensure mental healthcare accessibility to vulnerable and underprivileged sections of society. Despite its success in providing pharmacological interventions for MI, the delivery of psychotherapeutic interventions remains poor. Efforts have been made to address this issue with the introduction of the "Manpower Development Scheme", but the number of available clinical psychologists in public establishments is far less than the actual requirement (1.5 per 100,000).[34,35]

Ayushman Bharat (Universal Health Coverage scheme) provides coverage for mental health conditions. However, psychotherapeutic interventions have yet to be covered under the scheme. Most of the hospitals in the public sector are overburdened and need more qualified professionals to deliver psychotherapy.

Insurance schemes must cover psychotherapy for MI without discrimination, as envisioned by the Indian Mental Health Care Act, 2017.

Post-COVID, the need for mental health services has been emphasized, and there has been a rapid rise in the use of internet-based and telephone-based interventions. One significant advancement has been the Tele-MANAS program by the Government of India. This program aims to provide telephone services to people seeking mental health services with the option of call transfer to a psychiatrist/clinical psychologist when needed. Trained personnel provide this service, which includes counseling. The challenge would be maintaining the quality of services, and only briefer interventions would be feasible. This model needs to be tested for its fidelity and efficacy.

CONCLUSION

There is a considerable gap in the provision and availing of psychotherapy services in many LMICs, including India. Persons from low income-and illiteracy are at risk of developing CMDs, yet help-seeking rates are low.[36] The lack of trained mental health professionals to provide psychotherapy limits its usage. Attitudinal barriers of health professionals regarding the suitability of some forms of psychotherapy for the low-income individuals and illiterate even further widen the gap. If health is a fundamental human right, the treatment provisions should be equitable across all socioeconomic classes and literacy levels. When the basic needs are not met, the motivation to engage in psychotherapy, which can take time to show results, might be a challenge for the economically deprived. The way forward is to include psychotherapeutic skills training for all health professionals and the inclusion of psychotherapy as an available and acceptable treatment in guidelines for mental health problems.

REFERENCES

1. How many people live below the poverty line in India? It could be 34 million or 373 million. [online] Available from https://scroll.in/article/1048475/how-many-people-live-below-the-poverty-line-in-india-it-could-be-34-million-or-373-million [Last accessed December, 2023].
2. Visualizations. Government of India. [online] Available from https://censusindia.gov.in/census.website/data/data-visualizations/Literacy_Heatmap-Chart [Last accessed December, 2023].
3. Pabayo R, Fuller D, Goldstein RB, Kawachi I, Gilman SE. Income inequality among American states and the conditional risk of post-traumatic stress disorder. Soc Psychiatry Psychiatr Epidemiol. 2017;52(9):1195-204.
4. Lenart EK, Bee TK, Seger CP, Lewis RH, Filiberto DM, Huang DD, et al. Youth, poverty, and interpersonal violence: a recipe for PTSD. Trauma Surg Acute Care Open. 20211;6(1):e000710.
5. Shidhaye R, Patel V. Association of socio-economic, gender and health factors with common mental disorders in women: a population-based study of 5703 married rural women in India. Int J Epidemiol. 2010;39(6):1510-21.
6. Saraceno B, Barbui C. Poverty and Mental Illness. [online] Available from http://dx.doi.org/101177/070674379704200306. 1997 Apr 1;42(3):285–90 [Last accessed December, 2023].
7. Trani JF, Bakhshi P, Kuhlberg J, Narayanan SS, Venkataraman H, Mishra NN, et al. Mental illness, poverty and stigma in India: a case–control study. BMJ Open. 2015;5(2):e006355.
8. Patel V, Pereira J, Coutinho L, Fernandes R, Fernandes J, Mann A. Poverty, psychological disorder and disability in primary care attenders in Goa, India. Br J Psychiatry. 1998;172(6):533-6.
9. Wadsworth ME, Achenbach TM. Explaining the link between low socioeconomic status and psychopathology: testing two mechanisms of the social causation hypothesis. J Consult Clin Psychol. 2005;73(6):1146-53.
10. Banerjee S, Lev-Wiesel R, De S. Poverty, Somatisation Tendency and Potency in Low-Income Adolescent Groups of India and Israel: Explorations from the Field. Children. 2023;10(7):1104.
11. Ganga E, Chinyoka K. Exploring psychological disorders caused by poverty amongst orphans and vulnerable children living within child-headed households. Journal of sustainable Development in Africa. 2010;12(4):186-98.
12. Khattak T, Farooq S. Sociodemographic Features, Affective Symptoms and Family Functioning in Hospitalized Patients With Dissociative Disorder (Convulsion Type). J Pak Med Assoc. 2007;57(1):23-6.
13. Wendt FR, Pathak GA, Lencz T, Krystal JH, Gelernter J, Polimanti R. Multivariate genome-wide analysis of education, socioeconomic status and brain phenome. Nat Hum Behav. 2020 ;5(4):482-96.

14. Davis RG, Ressler KJ, Schwartz AC, Stephens KJ, Bradley RG. Treatment barriers for low-income, urban African Americans with undiagnosed posttraumatic stress disorder. J Trauma Stress. 2008;21(2):218-22.
15. Snell-Johns J, Mendez JL, Smith BH. Evidence-Based Solutions for Overcoming Access Barriers, Decreasing Attrition, and Promoting Change With Underserved Families. J Fam Psychol. 2004;18(1):19-35.
16. Jokela M, Batty G, Vahtera J, Elovainio M, Kivimäki M. Socioeconomic inequalities in common mental disorders and psychotherapy treatment in the UK between 1991 and 2009. Br J Psychiatry. 2013;202(2):115-20.
17. Briffault X, Sapinho D, Villamaux M, Kovess V. Factors associated with use of psychotherapy. Soc Psychiatry Psychiatr Epidemiol. 2008;43(2):165-71.
18. Epping J, Muschik D, Geyer S. Social inequalities in the utilization of outpatient psychotherapy: Analyses of registry data from German statutory health insurance. Int J Equity Health. 2017;16(1):147.
19. Bartram M, Stewart JM. Income-based inequities in access to psychotherapy and other mental health services in Canada and Australia. Health Policy (New York). 2019;123(1):45-50.
20. Hines-Martin V, Malone M, Kim S, Brown-Piper A. Barriers to mental health care access in an African American population. Issues Ment Health Nurs. 2003;24(3):237-56.
21. Gambrel P, Cianci, R. Maslow's hierarchy of needs: Does it apply in a collectivist culture? J Appl Manag Entrep. 2003;8:143-61.
22. Cooper-Patrick L, Gallo JJ, Powe NR, Steinwachs DM, Eaton WW, Ford DE. Mental Health Service Utilization by African Americans and Whites: The Baltimore Epidemiologic Catchment Area Follow-Up. Med Care. 1999;37(10):1034-45.
23. Diala CC, Muntaner C, Walrath C, Nickerson K, Laveist T, Leaf P. Racial/ethnic differences in attitudes toward seeking professional mental health services. Am J Public Health. 2001;91(5):805.
24. Mojtabai R. Americans' attitudes toward mental health treatment seeking: 1990-2003. Psychiatr Serv. 2007;58(5):642-51.
25. Du Plessis, Rory. Social class and psychotherapy: a critical reading of Thomas Szasz's the ethics of psychoanalysis. PINS. 2011;42:21-34.
26. Kazdin AE, Wassell G. Barriers to Treatment Participation and Therapeutic Change Among Children Referred for Conduct Disorder. J Clin Child Psychol. 1999;28(2):160-72.
27. Transforming Poverty-Related Policy with Intersectionality on JSTOR [Internet]. [online] Available from https://www.jstor.org/stable/44164853 [Last accessed December, 2025].
28. Borges AM. Psychologists' Experiences Working with Clients in Poverty: A Qualitative Descriptive Study. Boston College; 2014.
29. Kim S, Cardemil E. Effective psychotherapy with low-income clients: The importance of attending to social class. J Contemp Psychother. 2012;42(1):27.
30. Lenze SN, Potts MA. Brief Interpersonal Psychotherapy for depression during pregnancy in a low-income population: A randomized controlled trial. J Affect Disord. 2017;210:151-7.
31. Naeem F, Saeed S, Irfan M, Kiran T, Mehmood N, Gul M, et al. Brief culturally adapted CBT for psychosis (CaCBTp): A randomized controlled trial from a low income country. Schizophr Res. 2015;164(1–3):143-8.

32. Magidson JF, Gouse H, Psaros C, Remmert JE, O'Cleirigh C, Safren SA. Task Shifting and Delivery of Behavioral Medicine Interventions in Resource-Poor Global Settings: HIV/AIDS Treatment in sub-Saharan Africa. Massachusetts Gen Hosp Handb Behav Med; 2017.pp.297-320.
33. Kinyanjui DC, Ayuku DO. Task Shifting. Innov Glob Ment Heal. 2021;2:1287-301.
34. Khurana PH. National Mental Health Program of India: a review of the history and the current scenario. Int J Community Med Public Heal. 2016;3(10):2696-704.
35. Gangadhar BN, Kumar CN, Sadh K, Manjunatha N, Math SB, Kalaivanan RC, et al. Mental Health Programme in India: Has the tide really turned? Indian J Med Res. 2023;157(5):387.
36. Gururaj G, Varghese M, Benegal V, Rao G, Pathak K, Singh L, et al. National Mental Health Survey of India, 2015-16 Prevalence, Pattern and Outcomes; 2017.

5 CHAPTER How are We Treating the Suffering Children?

Vivek Agarwal, Chhitij Srivastava, Arundhati Gairola

ABSTRACT

The importance of psychotherapeutic approaches in India is on the rise due to the changing socio-cultural and economic structure of the society which has led to increasing stressors in modern life. This is especially relevant for children and adolescents because of concerns around safety of psychotropic medications. Various psychotherapeutic modalities are being practiced in India at limited places where trained manpower is available. Good evidence base for psychotherapy exists in the developed world but studies are limited in India and other low- and middle-income countries (LMICs). There is also huge variation in the practice of psychotherapy given the lack of standardized protocols. There are numerous other challenges in the practice of psychotherapy in India. This chapter will focus on the current evidence base of therapies in children, various challenges in the practice of psychotherapy in Indian population, and limitations of research.

Keywords: Psychotherapy, Children and adolescents, India, Evidence base

INTRODUCTION

Psychotherapeutic approaches play a vital role in addressing mental health issues. Their importance in India is on the rise due to the changing socio-cultural and economic structure of the society which has led to increasing stressors in modern life. As per the 2011 census, 40.69% of India's population is up to 19 years of age out of which about 12.5% suffer from diagnosable psychiatric disorders.[1] In children and adolescents (hereafter referred to as children unless specified), psychological interventions become especially important because of concerns around safety of psychotropic medications and paucity of research.

The western world has seen significant progress in the development of psychotherapies in children. Some of them are being practiced in India at limited places where trained manpower is available. This chapter will focus on evidence base of therapies in children, various challenges in practice of psychotherapy in Indian population, and limitations of research.

EVIDENCE BASE OF PSYCHOLOGICAL TREATMENTS

Problems of children can be broadly categorized as neurodevelopmental disorders like autism and learning disorders; externalizing disorders like oppositional defiant disorder; internalizing disorders like depression and anxiety disorders; severe psychiatric disorders like psychosis and bipolar disorders; substance use disorders, developing personality issues. Some adverse childhood experiences like child abuse and neglect deserve a special mention as they often play an extremely important part in the development of psychiatric disorders. Various psychotherapeutic interventions that have been found effective in these disorders using a parent or child approach have been summarized in **Table 1**.

TABLE 1: Summary of evidence-based psychological treatments for children and adolescents.

Psychiatric illness	*Psychological treatment*	*Reference*
Depression	• Cognitive-behavior therapy (CBT) • Interpersonal psychotherapy	• Asarnow et al. 2001[39] • Kaslow & Thompson 1998[40]
Anxiety disorders	• CBT • Systematic desensitization	• James et al. 2020[41] • Ollendick et al. 1998[42]
Obsessive compulsive disorder	CBT with ERP	Reid et al. 2021[8]
Oppositional/ conduct disorders	Parent management training (PMT)	Brestan & Eyberg 1998[43]
Autism spectrum disorder	• Applied behavior analysis (ABA) • Developmental models include DIR Floor time (The developmental, individual-differences and relationship-based model) and Naturalistic Developmental Behavioral Interventions (NDBIs) • Speech and language therapy (SALT) • Sensory integration therapy (SIT)	• Odom et al. 2010[44] • Solomon et al. 2014[45] • Schreibman et al. 2015[46] • Beukelman et al. 2005[47] • Case-Smith et al. 2015[48]
Attention-deficit/ hyperactivity disorder	PMT	Pelham et al. 1998[49]
Internet gaming disorder	CBT or multilevel counseling (MLC)	Chang et al. 2022[16]
Substance use disorder	Brief intervention including motivational interview	• Steele et al. 2020[50] • Li et al. 2015[51]
Tourettes syndrome	• Habit reversal training (HRT) • Behavior therapy including HRT and comprehensive behavioral • Intervention for tics	• Li et al. 2020[52] • McGuire et al. 2013[53]

A recent meta-analysis of 447 studies on various psychotherapies including 30,431 children demonstrated a moderate pooled effect size ($g = 0.46$) across treatments. When treating anxiety disorders, pooled effect size was largest (0.61), which was preceded by conduct problems (0.46), attention deficit/hyperactivity disorder (ADHD) (0.34) and depression (0.29).[2]

There is a lot of evidence for cognitive behavior therapy (CBT) in children. The effectiveness of CBT can vary depending on the actual process of therapy. For example, Whiteside et al., found larger effect sizes when in-session exposure and response prevention (ERP) had higher doses.[3,4] CBT has been successfully adapted to different disorders. Trauma focused cognitive-behavioral therapy (TF-CBT) for post-traumatic stress disorder (PTSD) is an excellent adaptation of CBT and had positive effects in trials conducted in various countries.[5-7] In the treatment of obsessive compulsive disorder (OCD), CBT with ERP had greater effectiveness than psychological placebo like psychoeducation ($g = 1.13$), and similar to CBT that focus largely on cognitive therapy ($g = 0.05$). Similarly, CBT with ERP had slight advantage over all forms of pharmacological treatment ($g = 0.36$).[8]

Meta-analyses of ADHD treatment trials have revealed mixed results, with behavior therapies showing most promising outcomes. However, in this group, the interventions are best provided through parents and teachers. Behavioral parent training and behavioral school-based interventions have pooled effect sizes of 0.70 and 0.66–0.72 respectively.[9] Miller & Lee's compiled 82 single subject experimental designs (SSEDs) studies comprising 168 participants with ADHD and concluded that functional analysis-guided interventions produced larger treatment effects.[10]

Psychotherapies for youth conduct problems yielded a pooled effect size of 0.82, according to Comer et al.[11] Aggression was found to have a significant overall small-to-medium effect size ($d = 0.28$) in multilevel meta-analysis. More effective interventions targeting the general population included behavioral practice and problem solving.[12]

Analysis of 44 randomized controlled trials (RCTs) reported dialectical behavioral therapies with reductions in self-harm (OR, 0.28) and suicidal ideation (Cohen *d* SMD, −0.71). Mentalization-based therapies were found effective in reducing self-harm (OR, 0.38) and suicidal ideation (Cohen *d* SMD, −1.22).[13] Studies that precisely evaluate treatments for nonepileptic seizures (NES) are scarce. It is not possible to draw a conclusion that one therapeutic technique was better than another from the existing literature, despite the fact that a variety of approaches have been used in managing conversion disorders with usually positive outcomes.[14]

According to recent research, psychosocial therapies like family-based therapy, CBT, and multicomponent approaches continue to be the most successful forms of treatment for adolescent substance use disorder.[15] A meta-analysis for treatment for Internet Addiction/Internet Gaming Disorder found that combining pharmacotherapy with CBT or multilevel counseling was the most effective treatment option.[16]

There is some evidence for efficacy of therapies done online. A meta-analysis of 37 RCTs on remote psychotherapies for youth on depression, anxiety, ADHD and conduct problems reported pooled effect size of 0.47 at post-treatment and 0.44 at follow-up that was comparable to results of meta-analyses of in-person youth psychotherapies.[17] However, the effect was significant for anxiety and conduct problems and not for depression and ADHD.

There is a wide range of sessions that are required for psychotherapy to be effective. The average number of sessions for youth psychotherapy examined in RCTs was 16, yet it was seen that young people only attend 1 to 4 sessions on average when receiving routine clinical care.[18,19] There were numerous RCTs evaluating single-session therapies as well. A meta-analysis of 50 RCTs of single-session therapy showed the average post-treatment impact size for all disorders was 0.32, with reasonable effects for anxiety (0.56) and behavior problems (0.54).[20] This study showed that it might be possible to do effective interventions in single session only.

EVIDENCE BASE IN LOW- AND MIDDLE-INCOME COUNTRIES

There is a huge gap when it comes to the evidence base of psychotherapies in low- and middle-income countries (LMICs). However, a recent meta-analysis with 43 treatment-control comparisons and 4,176 participants, showed pooled effects of youth psychotherapies in LMICs to be significantly larger than those in non-LMIC meta-analyses. However, the interventions that were culturally adapted from other nations had smaller effect sizes than those that were not. This probably means that in trying to adapt therapies to local cultures, there is a risk of altering the core therapy principles. An exception to this was evidence of successful application of culturally adapted DBT demonstrating that it is possible to adapt therapies effectively without modifying the fundamental principles.[21] However, there were high attrition rates in these trials as well as limited benefits of intervention by phone or by nonspecialist providers. Interventions delivered by the trained mental health professionals were more effective than lay persons. A systematic review of psychosocial interventions for self-harm in LMIC revealed that CBT and problem-solving therapy were the most extensively researched treatments.[22] Another meta-analysis targeting TF-CBT in LMIC showed it to be beneficial in addressing trauma-related symptoms and enhancing psychosocial functioning in children and adolescents.[23]

Parent/caregiver-mediated therapies make up the majority of autism intervention in LMIC (N = 8; 44%). Evidence suggests early intervention (ages 1–7) has beneficial effects on development.[24,25] However, the level of the evidence base is limited, with just a few successful replication studies.[26] In these studies, peer-mediated, parent-sibling-mediated as well as parent-teacher-mediated interventions were included. The periods ranged from 3 weeks to 6 months, with a wide range of the frequency of sessions (daily to weekly). There is some evidence that children with autism can benefit from interventions administered by nonspecialists in a variety of ways, particularly well-suited for LMICs.[27]

INDIAN RESEARCH

With respect to India, there is limited literature available on the effectiveness of psychotherapy in children. A review of interventions in ADHD of Indian studies reported efficacy of behavioral interventions in children.[28] Similarly, a study found manual-based parent skills training intervention for families having children with ADHD effective in reducing inattention, hyperactivity/impulsivity and conduct problems.[29] A computer-assisted CBT (Smartteen) in depression was noticeably more effective than TAU in improving depressive symptoms and functioning.[30] Another study reported efficacy of mindfulness-based cognitive therapy on children (MBCT-C) with anxiety.[31] Despite the paucity of data in India, the potential of therapy, along with its feasibility and acceptance, raises optimism for more research in this expanding field.

CHALLENGES IN PSYCHOTHERAPY PRACTICE

Providing psychotherapy to children in India presents a unique set of challenges that are influenced by cultural, social, and economic factors. Therapies which are being done are largely eclectic which involves exploration of stress, providing psychological support and possible resolution of stress or improving the coping skills. Therapies are usually not done as per manual. There are also numerous logistic challenges making it difficult to provide mental health services to those in need.

- *Lack of awareness and stigma:* In many parts of India, there is limited awareness about mental health issues as well as about the benefits of psychotherapy as a treatment option, leading to delayed or inadequate interventions. Stigma surrounding mental health issues remains prevalent in India, making it difficult for parents and caregivers to seek help for their children. Traditional cultural beliefs often attribute mental health issues to destiny or supernatural causes, which can deter families from seeking professional help. There is also a fear of negative social judgment and discrimination. Even when there is an acceptance of psychiatric illnesses, many Indian families especially from rural areas fail to see talking therapies as treatment modalities and seek medications instead.

- *Limited access to mental health services:* There is lack of availability of child psychiatric services in most parts of our country. Even if services of psychiatrist are available then clinical psychologist are not available so, the entire burden falls on the psychiatrist. As people come from distant places, it is not feasible for them to come frequently for therapy. Also, therapies are expensive other than the government sector and people find it difficult to afford. In government sector, therapists are few, leading to long waiting time or frequently missed appointments.
- *Training issues:* The therapy standards even in trained professionals can be very variable especially when it comes to the pediatric population. Most training institutes in psychiatry and psychology do not have a dedicated unit for the younger population which is a serious limiting factor. Besides, training in psychotherapy is also not very standardized with different institutes following different protocols. For example, in recent years, CBT has gained popularity in India as a valuable tool for addressing the emotional and psychological needs of children and adolescents. A recent review highlighted a number of pitfalls in the way CBT is being practiced in India.[32] These include incorrect interpretation of core CBT principles, using non-CBT techniques, side-lining cognitive aspect of CBT, etc. Some institutes are trying to adapt CBT to Indian context which alters the core CBT principles.

COMORBIDITY OF PSYCHIATRIC DISORDERS

There is a mismatch between the efficacy in clinical trials and effectiveness of therapy in community settings owing to the severe, comorbid conditions encountered in clinical practice. The rates of comorbidity are extremely high with around 40% of patients reporting more than one diagnosis comorbidity are extremely high with around 40% of patients reporting more than one diagnosis.[33] The high comorbidity rates probably do not represent true comorbidity but probably a shared common etiology between the reported comorbid disorders.[34,35] Current understanding shows that diagnostic boundaries are more fluid than previously believed and that it is important to focus on similarities between different disorders rather than focusing just on differences. Transdiagnostic treatments focus on shared common grounds between different diagnoses rather than the actual diagnosis and can address several comorbidities simultaneously. For example, a young person's eating disorder may be linked to her OCD symptoms. Rather than treating her eating disorder and OCD separately, they can be brought under one formulation based on the similarities and sometimes causal links and treatments can be designed to target both diagnoses simultaneously.[36] This has led to the development of Transdiagnostic CBT (TCBT) approaches to address symptoms and shared mechanisms across disorders. A recent Indian study found that such an approach can be successfully applied in our population.[37] Further it had the benefits of lowering costs and therapist time as it was targeting more than one disorder in a group setting. Another such approach termed "The PRIDE programme" is being piloted to develop transdiagnostic, low-intensity, stepped care psychological interventions addressing a wide range of emotional and behavioral problems among adolescents attending Government run secondary schools in India.[38] This is an exciting area in the practice of psychotherapy and is both an opportunity and a challenge in our population.

PRACTICAL PROBLEMS IN IMPARTING PSYCHOTHERAPY

Conditions in clinical trials are different from community settings with extensive pre-therapy training, close supervision on protocol adherence, and a small caseload of homogeneous clients. These ensure much better compliance than that can be seen in routine clinical practice. Even where trained personnel are available, it is difficult to ensure compliance to treatment protocols. Attrition rates are high as Indian families often look for quick results which psychotherapy does not provide. This means that therapies are often terminated midway with poor follow-up. A lot of therapies especially CBT involve home assignments that some children and their families are often reluctant to complete. Therapies are not always done in closed clinic rooms. However, most therapists do not extend therapy to outside clinic rooms because of workload, time constraints, traditional thinking about therapy. There are various other practical issues in providing therapy as explained below:

- *Communication barriers:* Communication with children poses its own set of challenges as children may not have the vocabulary or emotional awareness to express their feelings. Therapists need proper training to be able to communicate effectively with them using age-appropriate measures like play, stories, art, etc. A significant proportion of adolescents who are brought by their parents for help do not recognize any problem with their behavior. They do not see the need to seek help and therefore are reluctant to engage in therapy. Parents often resort to forcing them into the therapeutic process which makes the child-parent relationship worse. As expected, it leads to premature termination of therapy.
- *Child rights, consent and confidentiality:* Consent and confidentiality issues can arise when working with children, especially in cases where parents have differing opinions on the child's treatment. Often in Indian context, parents do not understand these issues and feel entitled to be made aware of all discussions that a young person has with the therapist.

This, therefore, makes it difficult for the young person to be able to trust the therapist and they become reluctant to share sensitive information with them often resulting in the failure of therapeutic process.

- *Family dynamics:* Traditional Indian families are joint families with multiple people in parenting role. While this is often an advantage, it also interferes with the therapeutic process with the young person who sometimes gets conflicting messages from different adults in the family. Family members also often hesitate to openly discuss relevant family dynamics which may be relevant to the therapeutic process. They may often also blame the child thus making it difficult for the therapist to come to a proper formulation and deliver effective therapy. Indian families also put a lot of emphasis on academic achievement of their children. While the focus on academics is a healthy thing, it can become excessive and almost feel like a burden that the child has to bear. Parents evaluate the outcome of therapy in context of academics.

LIMITATIONS OF RESEARCH IN PSYCHOLOGICAL TREATMENTS

Research in psychological treatments has not been able to provide moderators of treatment effects like characteristics of child or parents or culture, technique or effect of time. Similarly, it is not clear how the psychological treatments work. Studies have not been able to provide a consistent biological basis of effect of psychological treatments. Also, the treatments are largely focused on symptom reduction then overall recovery in different areas of impairment in the youth. Studies need to focus on these issues besides including children who are more similar to clinical settings to generalize the effects of therapies.

CONCLUSION

There is substantial evidence of efficacy of large number of psychological interventions in different disorders in youth. However, database in India is almost negligible. Reasons could be lack of mental health professionals, funding for research and overburdened professional with clinical care. The way forward may be use of technologies like app-based treatments, telemedicine as well as supervised treatment provided by trained lay persons. However, there is need to develop data base of effectiveness of interventions in Indian population to cater to the needs of huge population of youth.

REFERENCES

1. Srinath S, Girimaji SC, Gururaj G, Seshadri S, Subbakrishna DK, Bhola P, et al. Epidemiological study of child & adolescent psychiatric disorders in urban & rural areas of Bangalore, India. Indian J Med Res. 2005;122(1):67-79.

2. Weisz JR, Kuppens S, Ng MY, Eckshtain D, Ugueto AM, Vaughn-Coaxum R, et al. What five decades of research tells us about the effects of youth psychological therapy: A multilevel meta-analysis and implications for science and practice. Am Psychol. 2017;72(2):79-117.
3. Baker HJ, Lawrence PJ, Karalus J, Creswell C, Waite P. The Effectiveness of Psychological Therapies for Anxiety Disorders in Adolescents: A Meta-Analysis. Clin Child Fam Psychol Rev. 2021;24(4):765-82.
4. Whiteside SPH, Sim LA, Morrow AS, Farah WH, Hilliker DR, Murad MH, et al. A Meta-analysis to Guide the Enhancement of CBT for Childhood Anxiety: Exposure Over Anxiety Management. Clin Child Fam Psychol Rev. 2020;23(1):102-21.
5. Jensen TK, Holt T, Ormhaug SM, Egeland K, Granly L, Hoaas LC, et al. A randomized effectiveness study comparing trauma-focused cognitive behavioral therapy with therapy as usual for youth. J Clin Child Adolesc Psychol. 2014;43(3):356-69.
6. Murray LK, Skavenski S, Kane JC, Mayeya J, Dorsey S, Cohen JA, et al. Effectiveness of Trauma-Focused Cognitive Behavioral Therapy Among Trauma-Affected Children in Lusaka, Zambia: A Randomized Clinical Trial. JAMA Pediatr. 2015;169(8):761-9.
7. O'Callaghan P, McMullen J, Shannon C, Rafferty H, Black A. A randomized controlled trial of trauma-focused cognitive behavioral therapy for sexually exploited, war-affected Congolese girls. J Am Acad Child Adolesc Psychiatry. 2013;52(4):359-69.
8. Reid JE, Laws KR, Drummond L, Vismara M, Grancini B, Mpavaenda D, et al. Cognitive behavioural therapy with exposure and response prevention in the treatment of obsessive-compulsive disorder: A systematic review and meta-analysis of randomised controlled trials. Compr Psychiatry. 2021;106:152223.
9. Fabiano GA, Schatz NK, Aloe AM, Pelham WE, Smyth AC, Zhao X, et al. Comprehensive Meta-Analysis of Attention-Deficit/Hyperactivity Disorder Psychosocial Treatments Investigated Within Between Group Studies. Review of Educational Research. 2021;91(5):718-60.
10. Miller FG, Lee DL. Do Functional Behavioral Assessments Improve Intervention Effectiveness for Students Diagnosed with ADHD? A Single-Subject Meta-Analysis. J Behav Educ. 2013;22(3):253-82.
11. Comer JS, Chow C, Chan PT, Cooper-Vince C, Wilson LAS. Psychosocial Treatment Efficacy for Disruptive Behavior Problems in Very Young Children: A Meta-Analytic Examination. J Am Acad Child Adolesc Psychiatry. 2013;52(1):26-36.
12. Castillo-Eito L, Armitage CJ, Norman P, Day MR, Dogru OC, Rowe R. How can adolescent aggression be reduced? A multi-level meta-analysis. Clinical Psychology Review. 2020;78:101853.
13. Bahji A, Pierce M, Wong J, Roberge JN, Ortega I, Patten S. Comparative Efficacy and Acceptability of Psychotherapies for Self-harm and Suicidal Behavior Among Children and Adolescents: A Systematic Review and Network Meta-analysis. JAMA Netw Open. 2021;4(4):e216614.
14. Velani H, Gledhill J. The effectiveness of psychological interventions for children and adolescents with non-epileptic seizures. Seizure. 2021;93:20-31.

15. Fadus MC, Squeglia LM, Valadez EA, Tomko RL, Bryant BE, Gray KM. Adolescent Substance Use Disorder Treatment: An Update on Evidence-Based Strategies. Curr Psychiatry Rep. 2019;21(10):96.
16. Chang CH, Chang YC, Yang L, Tzang RF. The Comparative Efficacy of Treatments for Children and Young Adults with Internet Addiction/Internet Gaming Disorder: An Updated Meta-Analysis. IJERPH. 2022;19(5):2612.
17. Venturo-Conerly KE, Fitzpatrick OM, Horn RL, Ugueto AM, Weisz JR. Effectiveness of youth psychotherapy delivered remotely: A meta-analysis. Am Psychol. 2022;77(1):71-84.
18. Harpaz-Rotem I, Leslie D, Rosenheck RA. Treatment retention among children entering: A new episode of mental health care. Psychiatr Serv. 2004;55(9):1022-8.
19. McKay MM, Bannon Jr WM. Engaging families in child mental health services. Child and Child Adolesc Psychiatr Clin N Am. 2004;13(4):905-21.
20. Schleider JL, Weisz JR. Little Treatments, Promising Effects? Meta-Analysis of Single-Session Interventions for Youth Psychiatric Problems. J Am Acad Child Adolesc Psychiatry. 2017;56(2):107-15.
21. Haft SL, O'Grady SM, Shaller EAL, Liu NH. Cultural adaptations of dialectical behavior therapy: A systematic review. J Consult Clin Psychol. 2022;90(10):787-801.
22. Aggarwal S, Patton G, Berk M, Patel V. Psychosocial interventions for self-harm in low-income and middle-income countries: systematic review and theory of change. Soc Psychiatry Psychiatr Epidemiol. 2021;56(10):1729-50.
23. Thomas FC, Puente-Duran S, Mutschler C, Monson CM. Trauma-focused cognitive behavioral therapy for children and youth in low and middle-income countries: A systematic review. Child Adoles Ment Health. 2022;27(2):146-60.
24. Corsello CM. Early Intervention in Autism: Infants Young. Child. 2005;18(2):74-85.
25. Ben-Itzchak E, Zachor D. Who benefits from early intervention in autism spectrum disorders? Res Autism Spectr Disord. 2011;5:345-50.
26. McConachie H, Diggle T. Parent implemented early intervention for young children with autism spectrum disorder: A systematic review. J Eval Clin Pract. 2007;13(1):120-9.
27. Cherewick M, Daniel C, Shrestha CC, Giri P, Dukpa C, Cruz CM, et al. Psychosocial interventions for autistic children and adolescents delivered by non-specialists in low- and middle-income countries: a scoping review. Front Psychol. 2023;14:1181976.
28. Satapathy S, Choudhary V, Sharma R, Sagar R. Nonpharmacological Interventions for Children with Attention Deficit Hyperactivity Disorder in India: A Comprehensive and Comparative Research Update. Indian J Psychol Med. 2016;38(5):376-85.
29. Shah R, Sharma A, Grover S, Sachdeva D, Chakrabarti S, Avasthi A. Development and effectiveness of parent skills training intervention for Indian families having children with attention-deficit/hyperactivity disorder (ADHD). Asian J Psychiatr. 2021;64:102762.
30. Srivastava P, Mehta M, Sagar R, Ambekar A. Smartteen- a computer assisted cognitive behavior therapy for Indian adolescents with depression- a pilot study. Asian J Psychiatr. 2020;50:101970.
31. Shetty R, Kongasseri S, Rai S. Efficacy of Mindfulness Based Cognitive Therapy on Children With Anxiety. J Cogn Psychother. 2020;34(4):306-18.

32. Selvapandiyan J. Status of cognitive behaviour therapy in India: Pitfalls, limitations and future directions—A systematic review and critical analysis. Asian J Psychiatr. 2019;41:1-4.
33. Jacobi F, Höfler M, Siegert J, Mack S, Gerschler A, Scholl L, et al. Twelve-month prevalence, comorbidity and correlates of mental disorders in Germany: The Mental Health Module of the German Health Interview and Examination Survey for Adults (DEGS1-MH). Int J Methods Psychiatr Res. 2014;23(3):304-19.
34. Caspi A, Houts RM, Belsky DW, Goldman-Mellor SJ, Harrington H, Israel S, et al. The p Factor: One General Psychopathology Factor in the Structure of Psychiatric Disorders? Clin Psychol Sci. 2014;2(2):119-37.
35. Lahey BB, Moore TM, Kaczkurkin AN, Zald DH. Hierarchical models of psychopathology: empirical support, implications, and remaining issues. World Psychiatry. 2021;20(1):57-63.
36. Clark DA, Taylor S. The Transdiagnostic Perspective on Cognitive-Behavioral Therapy for Anxiety and Depression: New Wine for Old Wineskins? J Cogn Psychother. 2009;23(1):60-6.
37. Sharma P, Mehta M, Sagar R. Efficacy of transdiagnostic cognitive-behavioral group therapy for anxiety disorders and headache in adolescents. J Anxiety Disord. 2017;46:78-84.
38. Michelson D, Malik K, Krishna M, Sharma R, Mathur S, Bhat B, et al. Development of a transdiagnostic, low-intensity, psychological intervention for common adolescent mental health problems in Indian secondary schools. Behav Res Ther. 2020;130:103439.
39. Asarnow JR, Jaycox LH, Tompson MC. Depression in youth: psychosocial interventions. J Clin Child Psychol. 2001;30(1):33-47.
40. Kaslow NJ, Thompson MP. Applying the criteria for empirically supported treatments to studies of psychosocial interventions for child and adolescent depression. J Clin Child Psychol. 1998;27(2):146-55.
41. James AC, Reardon T, Soler A, James G, Creswell C. Cognitive behavioural therapy for anxiety disorders in children and adolescents. Cochrane Database Syst Rev. 2020;11(11):CD013162.
42. Ollendick TH, King NJ. Empirically supported treatments for children with phobic and anxiety disorders: current status. J Clin Child Psychol. 1998;27(2):156-67.
43. Brestan-Knight E, Eyberg S. Effective Psychosocial Treatments of Conduct-Disordered Children and Adolescents: 29 Years, 82 Studies, and 5,272 Kids. J Clin Child Psychol. 1998;27:180-9.
44. Odom SL, Boyd BA, Hall LJ, Hume K. Evaluation of comprehensive treatment models for individuals with autism spectrum disorders. J Autism Dev Disord. 2010;40(4):425-36.
45. Solomon R, Van Egeren LA, Mahoney G, Quon Huber MS, Zimmerman P. PLAY Project Home Consultation Intervention Program for Young Children With Autism Spectrum Disorders: A Randomized Controlled Trial. J Dev Behav Pediatr. 2014;35(8):475-85.
46. Schreibman L, Dawson G, Stahmer AC, Landa R, Rogers SJ, McGee GG, et al. Naturalistic Developmental Behavioral Interventions: Empirically Validated Treatments for Autism Spectrum Disorder. J Autism Dev Disord. 2015;45(8):2411-28.

47. Beukelman D, Mirenda P. Augmentative and Alternative Communication; 2012.
48. Case-Smith J, Weaver LL, Fristad MA. A systematic review of sensory processing interventions for children with autism spectrum disorders. Autism. 2015;19(2):133-48.
49. Pelham WE, Wheeler T, Chronis A. Empirically supported psychosocial treatments for attention deficit hyperactivity disorder. J Clin Child Psychol. 1998;27(2):190-205.
50. Steele DW, Becker SJ, Danko KJ, Balk EM, Adam GP, Saldanha IJ, et al. Brief Behavioral Interventions for Substance Use in Adolescents: A Meta-analysis. Pediatrics. 2020;146(4):e20200351.
51. Li L, Zhu S, Tse N, Tse S, Wong P. Effectiveness of motivational interviewing to reduce illicit drug use in adolescents: a systematic review and meta-analysis. Addiction. 2016;111(5):795-805.
52. Yu L, Li Y, Zhang J, Yan C, Wen F, Yan J, et al. The therapeutic effect of habit reversal training for Tourette syndrome: a meta-analysis of randomized control trials. Expert Rev Neurother. 2020;20(11):1189-96.
53. McGuire JF, Piacentini J, Brennan EA, Lewin AB, Murphy TK, Small BJ, et al. A meta-analysis of behavior therapy for Tourette Syndrome. J Psychiatr Res. 2014;50:106-12.

6 CHAPTER Placing Psychological Therapies in India in a Global Context

Neil Altman

ABSTRACT

In this chapter, I suggest that various versions of psychotherapy and psychoanalysis as they have evolved around the world reflect the local cultural context. To regard one version as "pure gold", to use Freud's characterization of the specifics of what he created in a European/Jewish context, itself reflects its colonial context. An exchange between Freud and Girindrashekhar Bose illustrates a counterproductive European dismissal of theoretical developments in India. Euro-American theorists began to accept some of Bose's points regarding gender only when these were framed as of Euro-American origin.

Keywords: Psychotherapy, Psychoanalysis, India, Colonialism, Bose

INTRODUCTION

Conventional wisdom has it that psychoanalysis is a foreign, western import, not really at home in India. I suggest alternative metaphors, based on the concept of "terroir", derived from the French word for soil, or earth, and referring more broadly to the way wine reflects the qualities of the land and the climate in which the grapes are grown and from which a given variety of wine is produced. This transplanted use of the word was introduced and applied to psychoanalysis by Mishra (Kumar, et al., 2018).

Psychoanalysis is a transplant, an immigrant, from European-Jewish soil, replanted in various terroirs around the world. In this chapter I consider what happens when psychoanalysis, bred to fit in the Viennese Jewish terroir is transplanted to the Indian terroir, then on to other parts of Europe, to North and South America and transplanted back again. Further, and more specifically, that the interaction between various versions of psychoanalysis and conditions of economic poverty varies widely between India and Europe/ North America, for example.

It is not commonly acknowledged that there has been a dialogue between European-bred psychoanalysis and Indian-bred psychoanalysis, raised amidst Indian ways of being and Indian ways of thinking since the early days of the field. Further, that the influence of India has always been detectable in the evolution of psychoanalysis elsewhere in the world, but under the radar, for the most part. The official history of psychoanalysis generally portrays the field as developing in Europe, then as Europe became inhospitable in World War ll, also in the parts of the Americas that received European refugees.

Meanwhile, India and Indians were making profound contributions to the field as if they amounted to a footnote in the official histories. Psychoanalytic marginalization of India paralleled a broader marginalization of India, its culture and its economy in the twentieth century British empire. An important part of the terroir in any given country is a function of colonialism and war.

BOSE

When institutional psychoanalysis, in the form of the International Psychoanalytic Association arrived in India, a challenge to Sigmund Freud's Oedipal theory emerged. Through 1920–1922, Girindrashekhar Bose of Calcutta, the first President of the Indian Psychoanalytic Society, and Sigmund Freud engaged in a correspondence in which Bose (1964) dissented from the idea of the Oedipus complex, a crucial weight-bearing pillar of Freudian theory. Bose's dissent, however, was essentially about gender. Bose claimed that Indians were less inclined to polarize masculinity and femininity, so that castration anxiety, arising from the male child's sexual attraction to his mother, was less threatening to Indian men than to European men. Freud insisted that castration anxiety along with the Oedipus complex were universal, always and everywhere the same. In footnotes (as in his Three Essays on Sexuality, 1905/1953), Freud put forward a more nuanced, less polarized, picture of gender, like that claimed as characteristically Indian by Bose. But Freud did not spell out the possible consequences of thinking of gender as having a less polarized structure. If gender has shades of gray, but if you also think of the critical marker of gender as the black-or-white presence or absence of a visible penis, then, of course gender identity as conventionally defined is always going to be tenuous for every boy. Bose (ignoring evidence of polarized conceptions of gender even in India) points out that if we take gender as nuanced, psychologically, despite the way anatomy (falsely) lends itself to either-or thinking, then the idea of universal castration anxiety universalizes childhood concrete thinking, along with one version of masculine psychology, common as that may be when reinforced by culture. If Freud had been more open to Bose's point, a great deal of feminist discrediting of psychoanalysis over the succeeding century might have been avoided. Why should the validity of psychoanalytic theory rise and fall on such flawed, culture-bound, reasoning?

WINNICOTT AND KHAN

India, represented by Bose, was up front on this point. His nonbinary view of gender was consistent with a long-standing tradition of nonbinary thinking in India on many fronts. For example, when foreign invaders arrived in India, the tendency was for their cultures to be assimilated into the Indian mainstream, rather than polarized and split off. Hinduism and Islam coexisted more or less peacefully for centuries in India until the collision with the British Empire with its insistence on supremacist domination. Ultimately, nationalism, a British/European import, was instituted in the form of the partition between India and Pakistan. Gray areas between Hinduism and Islam persist to this day in the form of Sufism which straddles the fence, even as Hindu supremacy prevails under the current Hindu nationalist regime. As late as the 1970s, in many households in India in which pictures of Hindu and Sikh deities lined the walls, space was made for a picture of Nehru and John F Kennedy walking together on a visit to India by JFK.

Bose's nonbinary view of gender thus fit within a long-standing Indian tradition, even when monotheistic Islam with its prohibition of religious iconography was added to the mix. But Freud was a monotheistic Jew, and European. At that moment there was no place for Bose's Indian nonbinary suggestion within Freud's psychoanalysis, so Bose's point of view remained marginal in the field until feminist critiques of patriarchal dominant/submissive structures found their way into psychoanalysis.

Meanwhile, however, DW Winnicott (1958) was, developing his own version of a nonbinary psychoanalysis as he, without much fanfare, replaced the idea of "contradiction" (either-or thinking) with "paradox" (both-and thinking). Winnicott was thus able to recast many core psychoanalytic concepts in the light of the notion of "transitional space", in which seeming opposites are seen to coexist. For example, in transitional space "fantasy" and "reality" can coexist. Our thinking about the nature of transference and countertransference are thus transformed. The space for thinking, accordion-like, is greatly expanded.

True to his nonbinary way, Winnicott never was inclined to an "out with the old", revolutionary, approach, to the steps in the evolution of psychoanalysis that he stimulated. For that reason I wrote above that Winnicott proceeded without "fanfare".

Nonbinary thinking found its way into Kleinian thinking as well in the form of developmental thinking based on "positions", as in "paranoid-schizoid" and "depressive" (Klein, 1975). Conceptions of development based on stages portray development as proceeding from one stage, step-wise, to the next stage. Stages are organized in a hierarchy, which lends itself to specific concepts of maturity and normality, a diagnostic framework with conceptions of pathology. Such a framework is not entirely absent from a "position theory", in the sense that one can still make judgments with respect to a proper balance between, say in paranoid-schizoid and depressive positions (remember that either-or thinking is in the background, but not eliminated). The point is that nonbinary thinking has major implications for developmental thinking as well as for thinking about transference and many other core psychoanalytic concepts. Winnicott did not use these differences to declare that a revolution was underway, much less to declare victory.

Where did Winnicott come up with his nonbinary way of thinking? I am intrigued by the fact that Masud Khan (Hopkins and Kuchuck, 2018) of Pakistani/Indian origin, was Winnicott's partner in innovation. I would not want to attribute the shape of Winnicott's thought to Khan, any more than I would be inclined to the opposite direction of influence. At the very least, there must have been a pre-existing receptivity in each to what the other had to offer, receptivity. Additionally, the South Asian-British chemistry contributed to shaping them both. Most analysts in the West take it for granted that Winnicott was the genius, the innovator, and that Khan was the follower, the editor of Winnicott's work. As pointed out above, however, Winnicott's work clearly has a large area of overlap with a South Asian sensibility, starting with the nonbinary framework, and including the definition of "true self" in terms of "going on being", an uninterrupted, unintruded-upon meditation-like flow of experience. Why should we assign priority to Winnicott in the generation of this picture of self, rather than to Khan, native to South Asia, perhaps carrying its sensibility in his bones? Do we unreflectively assign the dominant position to the colonizer, the submissive position to the colonized? Do we consider that perhaps Khan converted Winnicott to his way of thinking, or that Winnicott was unable or unwilling to credit Khan with having shaped his thought? Or, perhaps, we might consider that the situation was less linear, and that the particular alchemical product of this meeting of East and West, of psychoanalysis and Eastern spirituality, spontaneously combusted from the erotized dominant-submissive chemistry of Winnicott and Khan.

BION

If Winnicott was influenced by his intense experience with Pakistani Masud Khan, how much more did the spirit of India get into the psyche of Wilfred Bion (2018) who was raised in India, largely by an Indian nanny. She was the hands-on caregiver, while his parents kept their distance, ultimately sending him to a British boarding school.

In the next part of his life, he went to war, World War l, where he became a tank commander at age 16. At least in part from his experiences in the war, Bion developed a theory of trauma and the processes that allow for mental processing and growth when mental and emotional life have become frozen in the face of trauma. This theory became the basis for how Bion understood emotional development in infancy, and all through life, as well.

But Bion had been an infant and young child in India as well. There is an aspect of his view of early development that I think might have grown out of his immersion in, and absorption of, Indian culture as well via his nanny and other people. Bion recounts an anecdote in which, after returning from the war, his infant granddaughter was crawling toward him in the grass; Bion felt frozen, unable to reach out to her, position himself to pick her up. Bion identified this moment as the most painful in his life. Perhaps he was trying to support his granddaughter as his nanny had held and supported him. Instead he felt frozen and remote, far away like his mother.

Bion (1967) took a contrarian position with respect to mainstream psychoanalysis in "Notes on Memory and Desire". In this paper, Bion advocated that the analyst enter each session entirely in the here and now, divesting himself of any preconceptions about the analysand, or, indeed, about him- or herself. Bion thought that any preformed ideas about the patient or the process would prevent full openness to what was taking place here and now. Ram Dass (Richard Alpert) (1978) could not have said it more succinctly in his book "Be Here Now".

Bion went on to advocate that the analyst divest him or herself of desire, including the desire for cure or for the patient to change. This was a sharp break from a medical model of psychoanalysis, though close to Freud's "therapeutic pessimism". To fill out this idea, it might be more adequate to say that Freud's focus was on "research", i.e., to use clinical experience as data to develop and substantiate his psychoanalytic theory of psychopathology. He discovered, moreover, that his method of investigation, free association, with interpretation, had therapeutic effects. Research and therapy were both part of a unitary psychoanalytic process. Unlike other medical procedures, the investigation cured, at least some of the time.

There were occasions, however, when it became necessary to prioritize one or the other focus. In such cases, Freud tended to prioritize research, in the sense of theory development. Freud was self-critical (and criticized by others) for failing to interpret Dora's negative transference (Freud, 1905/1963). As a result, she dropped out of his research project, i.e., psychoanalysis. In a postscript, he realized that there was a negative transferential reaction that he had ignored. It did not seem to occur to him that there was an alternative understanding that would complicate his understanding of Dora's transference, i.e., that Dora felt Freud was exploiting her for his research, not unlike the way that Freud and her father were exploiting her to enable her father's affair with Frau K. She was offered up as a sexual object to Herr K in return for his not standing in the way of Dora's father's affair with Frau K. One might say that failing to understand Dora's situation in this way was consistent with the patriarchal norms of the time, but Freud steadfastly insisted that Dora's hysterical symptoms resulted from conflict over her sexual attraction to Herr K. If he had prioritized a cure, he might have named the exploitation and abuse to which teenage Dora was being subjected.

This is the aspect of Freud's technique to which Ferenczi (1933) objected, which later American interpersonalists (Levenson, 1978) referred to as "mystification". Ferenczi and others following him (e.g., Sullivan, Thompson) thought of such mystification as the primary pathogen, but this understanding was radically at odds with Freud's intrapsychic understanding which he was seeking to support in his presentation of the case of Dora.

Freud was led astray, in my view, by his commitment to a theory strongly biased toward the intrapsychic. But another understanding, more consistent with Bion's (1967) cautions about the pitfalls of desire, might have to do with the dangers of trying to fit square pegs into round holes in pursuit of some goal, e.g., whether that goal be to demonstrate his theory, even via a failure, or to support a theory via a successful cure, or some other narcissistically-fueled and inspired desire.

Thus far we have noted two points of controversy in psychoanalysis that split the field to a degree. One had to do with the priority given to the inner world, to internal objects as opposed to real people in the external world. The second had to do with the place of the analyst's subjectivity, in the form of desire, in the analytic field. Bions point is quite specific, having to do with the analyst's agenda, which he felt could shape or distort the analyst's openness to the previously unknown, or in some ways inherently unknowable, reality of the patient. The intrapsychic focus, along with the purism and nonutilitarianism which Freud and then Bion cultivated narrowed the appeal of psychoanalysis drastically. People will pay richly for purist, nonutilitarian activities, e.g., meditation classes, although it does not hurt if there is evidence that meditation lowers blood pressure. Nonetheless, if analysts pay little or no attention to the real world and if they do not aim primarily to help or cure, why pay them a lot of cold, hard, cash? It is a hard sell to convince insurance companies, which have a lot of power over the world of mental health these days, especially for the 99%, that they will save money by fostering widespread decreases in blood pressure by round about means, especially if there are pills available to do the same thing. And if you want the government to allocate taxpayers' hard earned cash to pay analysts, do not you have to produce evidence of demonstrable results in quantifiable (i.e., dollars and cents) terms? People only pay for more ephemeral results in the private sector, where contentment and such can serve as the coin of the realm. Thus, psychoanalysts gravitate toward the more affluent corners of the private sector, and the field becomes impoverished by turning away from the 99%, not to mention the (economically) poor. In the end, and ironically, that makes India an unlikely host for psychoanalysis.

There is a middle ground. There are psychoanalysts who try to make room in their practices for a number of affluent patients paying high fees while reserving some time for people who cannot pay so much (Vahali, personal communication, 1975).

Other analysts (e.g., Pine, 1988) recast theory and technique to fit what they consider the needs and capacities of "multiproblem families" (Pine, 1988) "Families of the Slums" (Minuchin, et al. 1967) or the "Urban Poor" (Altman, 2010). Sometimes adjustments are made in cases of "non-mainstream cultural backgrounds" or "minority" racial or language groups.

There is a danger in such cases of stereotyping people based on one aspect of their social status or identity. Sometimes what gets framed as an effort to be flexible amounts to a condescending assumption that people are incapable of the "real thing" as defined by psychoanalytic "criteria of analyzability". These efforts are typically well-intentioned and result on worthwhile work with people who might otherwise be more underserved.

Even as a marginal piece in the global mental health mosaic, psychoanalysis has made an important contribution, one that could be further extended and strengthened. Community-based work in war zones, with economically impoverished people, with refugees, exposes workers to vicarious trauma. People who choose such work find Bion's notion of containment, derived from his theory of how trauma can be processed and detoxified so one can go on living, invaluable. It is fitting that this product of Bion's life as a tank commander in World War I, including ways he found to go on living in the face of so much death, has been put to healing use.

GANDHI, KLEIN, AND BALDWIN

Mahatma Gandhi (Gandhi, et al., 1982) and Melanie Klein (1975) each produced innovative responses to the apparently endless vicious circles of violence in their worlds. In words sometimes attributed to Gandhi: "an eye for an eye leaves the whole world blind". Nonviolent resistance interrupts accelerating cycles of violence, defying the seeming inexorability of the death instinct. Klein's "projective identification" describes how disavowed destructiveness can be induced in other people, so that in the end, the destructive forces of which the projector wishes to be rid, appears to reside in others. Killing them can then seem justified in light of the danger that has been projected onto them. Frantz Fanon (1963) put this concept to use in describing how colonized people may identify with denigrated images of themselves in the eyes of their colonizers. Fanon built on Ferenczi's notion of "identification with the aggressor", which describes, in its original use, how the abused child identifies with the disavowed guilt of an abusive parent. Such occurs when sexually abused children are perceived as sexually seductive.

Klein, Fanon, Ferenczi, and Gandhi, all were looking for ways to interrupt self-reinforcing cycles of destructiveness. Each was trying to conceive, from the point of view of the seemingly powerless, of ways in which destructiveness could be contained, subject to thought, so that blind retaliatory destructive action could be interrupted or avoided.

An important supplement was added by James Baldwin (1993) the African-American novelist and minister, who detailed the spiritual and psychological price paid by the perpetrator of violent domination. Reading Gandhi in the past, I had reflected on how nonviolence seemed to be the perogative of the oppressed. The oppressor seemingly had nothing to gain from nonviolence since the violent oppressor would only lose what he had gained forcibly, since he could not forcibly defend it. Baldwin pointed out what the oppressor loses in perpetrating violence: his humanity.

Baldwin's premise was that vulnerability is an inevitable part of being human. The oppressor seeks the invulnerability promised by power and wealth, a false promise since we are all mortal, equally subject to sickness and death. If maturity is based on acceptance of reality, then to build a life based on false promises is a mark of immaturity. One can aim to be able to pay for the privileged life in a gated community far from the inner city rife with sickness and crime, but in the end, one is liable to be entrapped inside the gates of endless work hours and the anxiety of the vagaries of the stock market. One can aim to pay for the most expensive health care, precisely because one knows that one will need it, but hoping that the Fifth Avenue location of the doctor's office will provide some form of consolation.

Most fundamentally, one's privileges are purchased at the cost of dehumanization of others. The American dream of suburbia and exurbia is based on the fantasy that physical distance and locked gates can keep the reality of dehumanization and human vulnerability "out there". The frantic, manic search for more and more power and wealth exposes the subliminal knowledge that there's never enough, because the premise is a lie. Likewise, the stark discrepancies in power and wealth between countries, between the "global south" and the privileged "global north", the anxious exclusion of people migrating in search of a share in a "better life" exposes the shared conviction that privilege, "invulnerability", must be guarded at all costs by the dehumanization of others.

THE GLOBAL IMPACT ON THE SOCIO-ECONOMIC STATUS OF PSYCHOANALYSIS

As the Nazis came to power in Europe, Jews, including almost all the psychoanalysts in countries controlled by Nazis, were killed or forced to flee. Psychoanalysts took refuge in many countries throughout Europe and the Americas, especially England, the United States, and Argentina. Russell Jacobi (1986) described how psychoanalysis particularly in the United States, became a new home to emigre analysts.

Before the Nazi ascendancy, European psychoanalysts had been committed to social justice and leftist politics. Freud had called for free and low-cost psychoanalytic clinics throughout Europe. Such clinics sprung up throughout the continent (Danto, 2005).

As the analysts of Europe were expelled and dispersed around the world, an egalitarian vision survived in some quarters, particularly in Latin America. For example, Marie Langer, trained in Vienna, brought her social-psychoanalytic vision to Argentina, where she was a co-founder of the Argentine Psychoanalytic Association. Argentina was, and remains, a very active center of psychoanalytic thought, widely dispersed in society and engaged with the social world through the upheavals of military dictatorship and revolution of the 1970s and 1980s. Langer developed a psychoanalytically-oriented public mental health program in Nicaragua under the Sandinistas (Langer, 1989). The psychoanalysts of North America and Europe, remained unaware, or peripherally aware, of these developments.

Jacobi documented how in the United States, by contrast, the politics of psychoanalysts turned rightward. The United States had a long-standing capitalist tradition and an acute suspicion of the Soviet Union, it is formerly in World War ll, which was now in the hands of a Communist dictatorship. Psychoanalysts, largely noncitizens, were worried about being ostracized or deported if they were suspected of being Communists or communist sympathizers. Otto Fenichel and others, formerly active in leftist politics, went quiet.

Thus was reinforced a psychoanalytic withdrawal from the social-political world in the United States, one toward which psychoanalysis lent itself, with the intrapsychic orientation of its theory, and the degree to which its practitioners had been traumatized by the external world. A comfortable upper middle class status as private practitioners was appealing to these immigrants. For theoretical as well as political and historical reasons, psychoanalysis in the United States tended to set aside socio-economic origins to human suffering. Psychoanalytic fees were high, the clientele affluent, the public sector largely ignored and neglected. In Europe, this withdrawal from the social world was less extreme as psychoanalysts of England, for example, remained part of the public sector via the Tavistock Institute and the British National Health Service. This involvement with the public sector was productive of psychoanalytic engagement with people of lower socio-economic status and diverse ethnic origins. The prominent *Journal of Child Psychotherapy* is full of articles exploring the use to which psychoanalysis can be put in clinical work with foster children and their families, and in consultation with child care agencies and residential programs. Until recently, public funding of agencies with a diverse clientele in England stimulated psychoanalytic thought about how to take account of race, social class, and culture in clinical work. The Community Mental Health movement in the United States might have done the same, but has remained more peripheral to the North American psychoanalytic world.

INDIA

Meanwhile, India of the post-World War II years was preoccupied with efforts to free itself of the British Empire. The freedom struggle brought Mahatma Gandhi to prominence, highlighting his egalitarian and communitarian vision in sharp contrast to the individualistic focus of the United States. Nonetheless, among the multiple cultural cross-currents in Indian culture there were some points at which there was a potential fit between psychoanalysis and traditional Indian culture. For example, in Hindu culture, the guru-disciple relationship bears some points of overlap with the analyst-analysand relationship, both being intensively one-to-one, hierarchical, and aimed at the evolution of the analysand/disciple's spiritual/psychological development. In crucial respects, however, the Hindu/Buddhist spiritual and psychoanalytic/psychological realms are worlds apart, and there have been few efforts to bring them together (but see Ghent, 1990, Safran, 2003, for exceptions). Mindfulness, a concept derived from the discourse of meditation, has found a home in "wellness" practice, therapeutic without explicitly drawing on psychoanalysis.

PROSPECTS

In the remainder of this chapter, I develop my understanding of some deep commonalities between Gandhi's nonviolence and the cutting edge of Kleinian/Bionian psychoanalysis.

Finally, I elaborate on some ways I believe Indian culture, and evolving mental health practices in the area of community mental health have begun to feed each other.

Faced with the harsh realities of oppression, violence and war, Mahatma Gandhi developed the techniques and philosophy of nonviolent resistance. In the end, deployed with great commitment and intelligence, nonviolent resistance was key in getting the British out of India, perhaps in triggering the dissolution of colonial and racist domination around the world. Gandhi understood that violent resistance mostly was self-defeating. Nonviolent resistance provided more space not to be consumed by hatred and loss. Nelson Mandela, Archbishop Tutu, Lech Walesa, and Martin Luther King were inspired by Gandhi's vision to get out from under oppressive and violent domination by nonviolent resistance.

Meanwhile, in the context of World War, Melanie Klein developed her notion of the depressive position. World War I had led Sigmund Freud to develop his idea of a death instinct. Klein became occupied with the survival of goodness and love in the face of overwhelming destruction. The depressive position is a psychic space where goodness and badness can co-exist. In this sense, nonviolent resistance is enabled by the depressive position, violence is enabled by the paranoid-schizoid position where either goodness or badness dominates. The good kills off the bad, or vice versa.

The paranoid schizoid position enables passion and action. The depressive position enables complexity and thought.

Wilfred Bion took Kleinian thought forward with his elaboration of thought into "containment" through which mental life develops, integrating trauma.

Gandhi's power derived from his embodiment of both action and reflection. He was at once a political actor and a deeply spiritual person.

There have been others around the world who combined both of these qualities. Gandhi, however, was exceptional in his concern for the economically impoverished and for his egalitarian values. He renamed the castes which had been named "untouchable" with reference to their "unclean" occupations, such as cleaning toilets and disposing of dead bodies, "harijan", children of God. Nonetheless, some prominent harijans such as BR Ambedkar (2014) considered Gandhi as collusive with the caste system by even recognizing harijans as a group apart.

Gandhi's focus on the oppressed both carried forward and challenged an ancient Indian tradition of discrimination and oppression. Gandhi set an example of social consciousness that is recognizable in Indian psychoanalysis. This was not a country in which analysts could take refuge in comfortable ivory towers without being marginalized by their elitism.

Some years back, I received a Fulbright grant to help develop a training model for community-based psychoanalysis at Ambedkar University of Delhi (named after BR Ambedkar, mentioned above). The dean of the School of Human Studies, Honey Oberoi Vahali, and I planned to co-teach a class on Community Psychoanalysis. A few days before the class was to start, Honey called me into her office to say that she thought we, the faculty, later with our students, needed to get into the community, to have experiences with people who lived there from whom we would normally be insulated largely due to our own avoidance. Honey herself had a years-long relationship with a homeless family who lived on the street in Delhi. She knew from experience what was required to speak knowledgeably about psychoanalysis in the community. And so we did what she recommended. Here is an example of the kind of experience I had: (the following is excerpted from Altman, 2015, pp. 19-20).

Vignette 1

We, (faculty) along with the students, agreed to strike up a conversation with someone in a poor community that we would normally avoid, then to process the conversation in class with each other and the students.

As I was preparing to strike up such a conversation in a nearby market, I was taking a walk for exercise on a road that was in the process of being built for the Commonwealth Games in Delhi in 2010. Some high-rise buildings were being constructed to house the foreigners who were soon expected, and a new road was being prepared to make those buildings accessible. Construction workers lived in tents alongside the road. Women and men were breaking stones to cover the pavement while naked infants and barely clad children sat near them. There were latrines for these canvas encampments. As I passed by one such encampment, my eye was caught by a very thin man crossing the road with a tumbler of water in his hand, clearly planning to defecate in the field across the road rather than use the latrine. This method of defecating was once the norm all across India, but now the use of latrines is far more common.

As I passed by the encampment on my way back, I saw this man again on the side of the road. He had a baby on his hip, a little girl decked out in a pretty little dress and wearing black eye liner. The man, evidently her father, was coughing with a sound such as I had never heard. Directly on the baby. Later, I thought he must have had tuberculosis.

What I want to bring into focus is that as I passed this man, some one hundred feet away, I instinctively drew even further away from him all the way to the far edge of the road. There was no way I was close enough to catch whatever he had, but nonetheless, I needed to distance myself from him. Later, it occurred to me that my pulling away from him represented and enacted my anxiety about my forthcoming trip into a slum market. I, along with any other middle-class-and-up clinician preparing to enter a slum would be exposed to a range of diseases from which she would normally be protected and insulated. But, most of all, what seemed communicable was the suffering. How painful would it be to know that my beautiful baby girl was being exposed to the tuberculosis that I carried?

Looking back on this experience many years after the fact, I think the usefulness of going into the community as Honey suggested was not simply to experience the community but to experience what made us hitherto avoid the community, what anxieties were there, would always be there.

Vignette 2

One student in the class reported the following experience:

This student, a woman in her early twenties reported that she got into a rickshaw for a short trip. The driver was a man in his mid-forties. "Rickshaw drivers often talk to me, so I thought this would be a good opportunity for me to have a conversation," reported this open-faced young woman. As the rickshaw moved along in fits and starts in the heavy traffic of Delhi, the driver would turn around when there was a short stop to say something to his passenger. At the first stop, he said, "I have a son and a daughter and a computer". The student said nothing. At the next stop he said: "And I found my son watching one of 'those movies' on the computer". Again, the student said nothing, just listened. At the next opportunity, the driver said "I guess he's getting to the age where he's having 'those desires'. And then, "I guess my daughter is having those desires, too", to which the student said "May be so". At the next stop he said "I have those desires" and then a question: "Do you have those desires?". To which she responded "Not yet". And then "Not since my mother died 2 years ago". Nearing their destination, the driver then said "My wife and I didn't know anything about sex when we got married, but we've learned that sex is a very important part of a marriage". At which point, the destination reached, the conversation was over.

In the discussion of this conversation in the class, another student asked what was on everyone's mind "Were you scared?" To which the student replied "At one point I wondered if I should be scared, but actually I wasn't".

My own conclusion is that this conversation was a kind of therapy session. The driver, finding a receptive listener, brought a problem: how to deal with his son's emerging sexuality in the age of the internet. He found a daughter-type person who set limits ("not yet" she said about her own desires) while opening herself up in a personal way about the death of her mother and its impact on her own sexuality. With this frame in place, he could have a safe and straight forward conversation with her, about sex, an experience that presumably will facilitate his ability to have a discussion with his children.

In order to regard this conversation as a "session", a "psychoanalytic" session, we must be flexible about definitions. There was no office other than the rickshaw itself. There was no time boundary other than the length of the ride. The fee was on the meter. Yet if psychoanalysis is defined, per Freud, as the analysis of resistance and transference, all the ingredients are there in this vignette. The frame provided by the rickshaw trip was perfect for eliciting the driver's unconscious sexual concern in the context of the relationship with the student/analyst.

The therapeutic potential in such exchanges has been harnessed by Vikram Patel (2002) who has developed a community-based project called "Sangath". Paraprofessionals and laypersons from the community are trained to identify depressed people in their own community, to have conversations with them in their homes or in medical doctors' office where they might come with somatic complaints. This is an example of an approach that reaches people where they are, that might build on concerns ("somatic") that they already have, in conversations (sessions) with people they trust (from their own community).

CONCLUSION

Recent years have brought trends that support East-West and North-South communication and sharing in psychoanalysis and other fields. Past obstacles to such cross fertilization include colonialism that has led to dismissal and denigration of contributions from the "developing" world. The fact is that all parts of the world are developing and all can learn from each other. We need to think together as well to make sure that psychoanalytic therapy is available to as many people as possible in culturally accessible ways.

FURTHER READING

1. Altman, N. Psychoanalysis in an Age of Accelerating Cultural Change: Spiritual Globalization. New York and London: Routledge; 2015.
2. Altman, N. The Analyst in the Inner City: Race, Class, and Culture through a Psychoanalytic Lens, second edition. New York and London: Routledge; 2010.
3. Ambedkar BR. Annihilation of Caste. London and New York: Verso; 2014.
4. Baldwin J. The Fire Next Time. New York. Vintage International; 1993.
5. Bion WRD. Notes on memory and desire. 1967;2:272-3, 279-80.
6. Bose G. The Beginnings of Psychoanalysis in India: The Bose-Freud Correspondence. Calcutta: Indian Psychoanalytical Society; 1964.
7. Danto E. Freud's Free Clinics: Psychoanalysis and Social Justice, 1918-1928. New York: Teachers College Press; 2005.
8. Fanon F. The Wretched of the Earth New York: Grove Press; 1963.
9. Ferenczi S. Confusion of tongues between the adults and the child (the language of tenderness and of passion). Int J Psychoanal. 1933;30:225-230.
10. Freud S. Beyond the pleasure principle. In: J Strachey (Ed). The Standard Edition of the Complete Psychological Works of Sigmund Freud. London: Hogarth Press. 1920;18:1-64.
11. Freud S. Dora: An Analysis of a Case of Hysteria. New York; Grove Press; 1905/1963.
12. Freud S. Three essays on the theory of sexuality. In: J Strachey (Ed). The Standard Edition of the Complete Psychological Works of Sigmund Freud. London: Hogarth Press. 1905/1953;7:125-245.
13. Gandhi M, Gandhi MK, Das V. An Autobiography: The Story of My Experiments with Truth. Delhi: Navajivan; 1982.
14. Ghent E. Masochism, submission and surrender: masochism as a perversion of surrender. Contemporary Psychoanalysis. 1990;26:108-36.
15. Hopkins L, Kuchuck S. Psychoanalysis. Diary of a Fallen Psychoanalyst: The Work Books of Masud Khan 1967-1972. London: Karnak; 2022.
16. Jacobi R. The Repression of Psychoanalysis: Otto Fenichel and the Political Freudians. Chicago/London: University of Chicago Press; 1986.
17. Klein M. Love, Guilt, and Reparation and Other Works 1921-1945. New York: Delta; 1975.
18. Kumar M, Dhar A, Mishra A. Psychoanalysis from the Indian Terroir: Emerging Themes in Culture, Family, Childhood. Lanham, MD: Lexington Books; 2018.
19. Langer, M. From Vienna to Managua: Journey of a Psychoanalyst. London: Free Association Press; 1989.
20. Levenson E. Two essays in psychoanalytic psychology: I: Psychoanalysis: cure or persuasion? Contemporary Psychoanalysis. 1978;14(1):1-17.
21. Minuchin S, Montalvo B, Guerney BG, Rodman BL. Families of the Slums: An Exploration of Their Structure and Treatment. New York: Basic Books; 1967.

22. Patel V. Where There is no Psychiatrist. London: Gaskell; 2002.
23. Pine F. Developmental Theory and Clinical Process. New Haven, CT; Yale University Press; 1985.
24. Ram Das B. Be Here Now. Easton, PA: Harmony Press; 1978.
25. Safran J. Psychoanalysis and Buddhism: An Unfolding Dialogue. Somerville, MA: Wisdom Press; 2003.
26. The Long Weekend 1897-1919: Part of a Life. London and New York: Routledge; 2018.
27. Winnicott DW. Transitional objects and transitional %phenomena. In: Collected Papers: Through Pediatrics to Psychoanalysis. New York: Basic Books; 1958. pp. 229/2242.

SECTION 2

Helpful Echoes from the Indian Diaspora

7

CHAPTER

Psychotherapy in the Sacred Hindu Text: The Bhagavad Gita

Satish Reddy

ABSTRACT

In this contribution, the Bhagavad Gita is approached as a psychoanalytic discourse. The dialogue between Arjuna and Lord Krishna is seen as a psychotherapeutic process, replete with resistances, transferences and cognitive distortions. Arjuna's inhibition to fight is precipitated by the Oedipal guilt of killing paternal surrogates, Bhishma and Drona. The sensory modality of vision is central to Arjuna's spiritual conversion and his identification with Krishna as God. The overwhelming feelings of awe, wonder and fear of seeing Krishna as God figure prominently in Arjuna's conversion. The Hindu ritual of a Darshan is compared to Arjuna's vision of God in chapter 11 of the *Gita*. The implications of these proposals for the conduct of psychotherapy are elucidated.

Keywords: Bhagavad gita, Psychotherapy, Psychotherapeutic process

INTRODUCTION

The Bhagavad Gita (Gita), literally meaning "The Song of God", is one of the most sacred texts of Hinduism. It is a part of the great Sanskrit epic, "The Mahabharata". The *Gita* is a conversation between the god Krishna and his human pupil Arjuna. Composed around 200 BC, the *Gita* is a profound document. It outlines the Hindu position on the nature of the body and soul, man's duty on earth and the path to salvation. It is a beautiful synthesis of the core concepts of Hinduism. It is also one of the earliest recorded documents of psychotherapy.

The *Gita* is set in the context of an apocalyptic fratricidal war. Arjuna is the epic warrior hero and Krishna is his chariot driver. Unaware of Krishna's divinity, Arjuna thinks of him as his close friend. Before the war begins, Arjuna is overwhelmed by sadness at the prospect of killing his relatives and friends. He tells Krishna that he will not fight. Paralyzed by guilt and fear, Arjuna asks for Krishna's help. Krishna's counsel to Arjuna comprises the core content of the Gita. In its eighteen dense and terse chapters, Krishna conveys to Arjuna the essential teachings of Hinduism and provides a path for Arjuna to overcome his existential crisis. In chapter 1, Arjuna tells Krishna "I will not fight". At the end of the *Gita*, in chapter 18 , he tells Krishna: "Here I stand with no more doubts. I shall do as you say." (*Gita* 18:70)

The discourse of the *Gita* can be seen as a transformative dialogue, that while culturally and idiomatically distinct, is akin to psychotherapeutic process. Following Hans Loewald:

> "By psychoanalytic process I mean the significant interaction between patient and analyst that ultimately leads to structural changes in the patient's personality...If structural changes in the patient's 'personality' means anything, it must mean that we assume that ego development is resumed in the therapeutic process in analysis. And this resumption of ego development is contingent on the relationship with a new object, the analyst". (Loewald, 1960, p.16).

In the *Gita,* Krishna functions as Arjuna's teacher (*Guru*) and I propose as his psychotherapist. Krishna's therapeutic function is not interpretive but more as an object that facilitates Arjuna's psychic-ego development. Specifically, Krishna allows Arjuna to use him as a transformational object. The transformational object, by eventuating a transformation, becomes sacred, an object of *Bhakti,* a uniquely Hindu form of devotion. From a psychoanalytic view, the cardinal techniques of anonymity, abstinence and neutrality are both observed and violated by Krishna. But the pivotal violation of anonymity in chapter 11, by Krishna's self-disclosure as God, promotes the therapeutic regression and psychic reorganization that leads to Arjuna's existential transformation.

THE STRUCTURE AND LOGIC OF THE GITA

The *Gita* is a small part of the vast Hindu epic, *The Mahabharata,* a text of about 75,000 verses. The *Mahabharata* is the story of a great eschatological war between the five Pandava brothers and their cousins, the 100 Kauravas, who are fighting for dominion over a kingdom. This complex and fascinating text consists of 18 major books (*parvans*), each subdivided into chapters. The chapter entitled "The Book of the Bhagavad Gita" is located in the sixth major book, *Bhismaparvan,* named after Bhishma, great grandfather and patriarch to both warring parties. This book chronicles the killing of Bhishma by Arjuna. The central plot of the *Mahabharata* revolves around Bhishma's voluntary renunciation of his father's throne and his vow of lifelong celibacy so that his father may marry a low caste woman. Bhishma's Oedipal submissive actions result in problems to the royal succession, culminating in the war between the Pandavas and the Kauravas.

The *Gita* is a short treatise: 600 stanzas divided into 18 chapters. It is narrated as a poetic dialogue between the bard Sanjaya and his patron, the blind king Dhrtarastra, father of the Kauravas. Sanjaya has been given the gift of telepathy, and is relating the details of the war to the blind king at his palace.

The first 10 chapters consist of Arjuna's crisis and Krishna's attempts at resolving it. Chapter 2 contains the core teaching of the *Gita*. If Arjuna understood what Krishna was saying in chapter 2, the rest of the *Gita* would be unnecessary. However, Arjuna's resistances are powerful and lead to Krishna's continuation of his teaching. Chapter 11 is the pivotal chapter where Arjuna undergoes a profound psychic regression and metamorphosis through a vision of Krishna's divinity. The transference is one of fear and awe. Chapter 11 is the fulcrum on which the *Gita* oscillates. When Arjuna asks Krishna who he is, Krishna responds, "I am time grown old to destroy the world". (*Gita*: 11:32). Chapter 11 negates, transcends, and collapses chronological time and takes us into Krishna's divinity and timelessness.

Chapters 12–18 are a continuation of Krishna's teaching, but with a difference. Arjuna has gained insight. He is at a higher grade of ego development and maturation. Arjuna's development of *Bhakti* (devotion) becomes a prominent theme. Krishna, the charioteer and friend, becomes an object of devotion. Krishna, the transformational object, becomes the sacred object. Arjuna's questions and doubts remain but at a higher level of awareness and consciousness. Each stage is replete with its corresponding resistances, transferences, and cognitive distortions. Chapters 1–10 are heavily intellectual. Chapter 11 is uniquely mystical. Chapters 12–18 develop *Bhakti*, the uniquely devotional aspect of Hinduism.

KURUKSETHRA: THE BATTLEFIELD AS THE PSYCHOTHERAPEUTIC SETTING

The first stanza of the *Gita* reads:

"When in the field of the Kurus, the Field of the Law, my troops and the Pandavas had massed belligerently, what did they do, Sanjaya?" (*Gita* 1, 1)

The setting of the *Gita* is the battlefield. The *Gita's* occurrence in the "middle" of the battlefield is noteworthy, as middle connotes neutrality. The middle or center is a neutral place to observe and contemplate action. Middle connotes not only neutrality but also equidistance of intrapsychic domains vying for dominance. Anna Freud comments on this notion by her recommendation that technically and ideally, the analyst should be positioned equidistant from the analysand's id, ego and the superego. (Anna Freud, 1966)

The middle or center characterizes Krishna's perspective. He is centered and grounded within himself, neutral and impartial, both to himself as the agent of the action and to the result of the action. This is the doctrine of selfless action, known as *Karma Yoga*. In contrast, Arjuna is not centered. He identifies himself as the agent of the action. His identifications, the root cause of his problems, lead to his dejection, pity and inability to act. Krishna says:

> "Your entitlement is only to the rite, not ever at all to its fruits. Be not motivated by the fruits of the acts, but also do not purposely seek to avoid acting. Abandon self-interest, Dhananjaya, and perform the acts while applying this single mindedness. Remain equable in success and failure—this equableness is called the application, for the act as such is far inferior to the application of singleness of purpose to it." (*Gita*, 2, 48–49)

It is significant that the *Gita* occurs in the battlefield. *Kurukshetra* refers not only to the literal battlefield but metaphorically to Arjuna's intrapsychic and interpersonal battlefield. In contrast to the calm setting of the analytic office with the patient lying on the couch, the dialogue between Krishna and Arjuna occurs in a chariot positioned between two hostile armies, amidst all the noise and clamor. Freud, in his *Outline of Psychoanalysis*, likened the analytic situation to a civil war:

> "The ego is weakened by the internal conflict and we must go to its help. *The position is like that of a civil war which has to be decided by the assistance of an ally from the outside.* The analytic physician and the patient's weakened ego, basing themselves on the real external world, have to band themselves together into a party against the enemies, the instinctual demands of the id and the conscientious demands of the superego. We form a pact with each other. The sick ego promises us the most complete candor-promises, that is, to put at our disposal all the material which its self-perception yields it; we assure the patient of the strictest discretion and place at his service our experience in interpreting material that has been influenced by the unconscious. Our knowledge is to make up for his ignorance and give the ego back its mastery over lost provinces of his mental life. *This pact constitutes the analytic situation*" (Freud, 1940, p.173, italics mine)

It is not the quietness and distraction from external stimuli that defines the psychotherapeutic setting but rather the capacity of the analyst to create a safe "holding environment" (Winnicott, 1960). In the hostile and dangerous space between two warring armies, Krishna creates the safe "holding environment" where Arjuna's transformation occurs.

THE CONTEXT OF THE GITA

The *Gita* occurs in the 6th book of the *Mahabharata, The Bhishmaparvan* (*Book of Bhishma*), in a chapter entitled *The Bhagavadgitaparvan* (*The Book of the Bhagavadgita*). Bhishma is great grandfather and patriarch to both warring parties and a celebrated hero and warrior from previous generations. He becomes the first general of the Kaurava army. *The Book of Bhishma* chronicles the killing of Bhishma by Arjuna. It is the thought of killing Bhishma that precipitates Arjuna's crisis.

The Book of the Bhagavadgita begins with the announcement by Sanjaya to his patron, the blind king Dhritarashtra (father of the Kauvaras) that Bhishma has fallen in battle. Dhritarashtra is stunned by the news. He questions Sanjaya how this happened. The *Gita* occurs midway in the *Book of the Bhagavadgita.* Its positioning here in the epic is psychologically important: "It is not just a successful narrative device that the death of Bhishma is first reported as an accomplished fact, then juxtaposed with the prior teaching of the *Gita* which in the end seeks to justify the killing of him: each one is the condition of the other." (Van Buitenen, 1980, p.1) Chronologically, before the *Gita* begins, Arjuna has already slain Bhishma. The dialogue of the *Gita* begins *ex post facto:*

> "The preamble tells us that Bhishma is dead, that Arjuna's reluctance to fight in this war was therefore fully justified, and that consequently a need existed to override Arjuna's reluctance with a higher truth, so that in fact *that* will come about which we know is *already* the case." (Van Buitenen, 1980, p.3)

WHO IS KRISHNA?

In the *Mahabharata*, Krishna fluctuates between the human and divine, similar to Christ in the New Testament. Krishna is Arjuna's cousin and close friend. "Of the Pandavas, Arjuna was the same age as Krishna. He always bowed to Dharma (his eldest brother) and Bhishma as his elders, and was, in turn, shown respect by the twins (his youngest brothers), but he always embraced Krishna as his equal. These two picnicked together, drank together, and were intimate friends." (Karve, 163). Krishna is also a warrior and an epic hero himself—a king of the Yadava clan. His identity in the epic can be confusing, perhaps intentionally so by the authors. Krishna is human to most, recognized as divine by a few, and revealed as God to one. His sympathies and affinity are with the Pandavas, particularly Arjuna. In the *Mahabharata*, Krishna offers his army to one side and his presence as a noncombatant in the war to the other side. Arjuna chooses Krishna's presence while Duryodhana (the Kaurava king) chooses Krishna's army. Duryodhana is pleased with the arrangement that he has Krishna's formidable army—a better deal than having Krishna's presence. Duryodhana thinks of Krishna as another king with a powerful army vying after his own self-interest. Arjuna, on the other hand, is delighted to have his close friend and soul mate Krishna as his chariot driver. Did Arjuna have an unconscious inkling that Krishna was more than he appeared?

> "Who then is Krishna who persuades Arjuna to accept the warriors fate? He is a *Vrisni* prince, for the nonce acting as Arjuna's charioteer, a seemingly subordinate role to which he has agreed in order to be a noncombatant in the thick of battle. Loyal to both warring parties, he has conceded his troops to Duryodhana and his presence to Arjuna... This role assumed by Krishna, because of the conventional camaraderie between warrior and driver, provides the intimacy which makes his exhortations possible and appropriate. Traditionally, the *suta* (chariot driver), on the chariot of the warrior, is witness to the warrior's triumphs and occasional lapses; in danger, he protects him. The triumphs of the warrior, he celebrates in song, hence *suta* also means bard. The lapses he condemns in private." (van Buitenen, p.4-5)

Krishna is importantly an *avatar* of God— in Hinduism, a descent of God into man or God coming down to earth to re-establish morality and order. An *avatar* is a voluntary and deliberate act of God.

> "For whenever the law languishes, Bharata, and lawlessness flourishes, I create myself. I take on existence from eon to eon, for the rescue of the good and the destruction of the evil, in order to reestablish the law". *(Gita,* 4:7-8)

■ ARJUNA'S CRISIS: THE SICK AND DIVIDED SELF

Arjuna's crisis is vividly described in chapter 1 of the *Gita*. As war is about to begin, Arjuna asks Krishna to place his chariot between the two armies. Arjuna sees in both armies his family, friends, and teachers. He becomes sad and despondent:

> "Krishna, when I see all my family poised for war, my limbs falter and my mouth goes dry. There is a tremor in my body and my hairs bristle. Gandiva (celestial bow) is slipping from my hand and my skin is burning. I am not able to hold my ground and my mind seems to whirl. And I see contrary portents, Kesava, but I see no good to kill my family in battle! I do not wish victory, Kesava, nor kingship and pleasures. What use is kingship to us, Govinda? What use are comforts and life? The very men for whose sake we want kingship, comforts, and joy, stand in line to battle us, forfeiting their hard to relinquish lives. Teachers, fathers, sons, grandfathers, maternal uncles, fathers-in-law, grandsons, brothers-in law, and other relatives-in-law—I do not wish to kill them though they be killers, Madhusudana, even for the sovereignty of the three worlds, let alone earth." (*Gita*, 1, 29-32)

Note the dejection, guilt, anhedonia and hopelessness in Arjuna's words. He is displaying the classic symptoms of melancholic depression. Arjuna drops his *Gandiva* bow and sits dejected and helpless in his chariot saying that he will not fight.

It is important to note that in a text as short and succinct as the *Gita*, a whole chapter is devoted to Arjuna's despondency. From a psychoanalytic view, Arjuna's inhibition to fight and his depression are precipitated by Oedipal guilt-specifically the killing of Bhishma, the *paternal figure par excellence* and Drona, Arjuna's teacher and *guru* (another crucial Oedipal object). Bhishma, the supreme commander of the Kaurava army, is loved and revered by Arjuna. They have grown up in the same house and a special affection and bond develops between them. It is not coincidence that the *Gita* is located in the "Book of Bhishma". Its positioning there reflects and emphasizes the Oedipal dynamics of patricide and guilt, and explains Arjuna's profound ambivalence about fighting and killing Bhishma.

> "How, Krishna, shall I fight in battle, with the venerable and aged preceptor of the Kurus, the grandsire of accomplished understanding and intelligence? Krishna, while playing in the days of childhood, I used to soil the garments of the high souled and illustrious one by climbing on his lap with my body smeared with dust. Krishna, in my childhood, climbing on the lap of the high souled father of Pandu (our father), I used to say 'father'. 'I am not your father, but your father's father, Arjuna, were the words he used to say in reply to me. Oh how he used to treat me thus; how could he be now slain by me." (*Mahabharata*, Book 6, chapter 108, verses 90-93)

A closer look at the first chapter shows us that Arjuna not only questioned his morality in killing, but also Krishna's morality when the latter repeatedly prompts him to kill Bhishma.

> "Arjuna's dilemma is a real one and, despite Krishna's sarcasm, an honorable one. In effect, on the level of *dharma* (duty), Arjuna will be proved to have been right; but in the *Gita* Krishna offers him the choice of another level of values, which will absolve him from guilt." (van Buitenen, p.3)

Arjuna's depression is an important and necessary condition for his spiritual conversion. His "battlefield paralysis", his neurasthenia, goes far beyond the moral questioning of war. It reflects a deeper spiritual crisis. As a warrior, Arjuna had fought and killed many times before-without remorse or guilt. This was his "profession"-his *Dharma* or duty in life as defined by the Hindu caste system. A role at which he excelled and indeed, was considered incomparable. It is implausible that moral doubts about killing alone paralyzed Arjuna. It was guilt over slaying parental surrogates and teachers ("*gurus*") that lead to him questioning his self and his moral duty.

William James posits that such a guilty sense of "sin" is prerequisite for spiritual conversion.

> "To begin with, there are two things in the mind of the candidate for conversion: first, the present incompleteness or wrongness, the 'sin' which he is eager to escape from; and, second, the positive ideal which he longs to compass. Now with most of us the sense of our present wrongness is a far more distinct piece of our consciousness than is the imagination of any positive ideal we can aim at. In a majority of cases, indeed, the 'sin' almost exclusively engrosses the attention, so that conversion is a process of struggling away from sin rather than of striving towards righteousness." (James, p.187)

As James notes, a necessary condition for spiritual conversion is a self that is plagued by guilt about what it has done or what it is going to do rather than a narcissistic self-aiming to prefect itself. Negative and painful emotions motivate men to seek spirituality and other worldly reassurances. The comfortable are poor candidates for spiritual conversion.

Arjuna's problem was that he did not know how to act. Specifically, should he fight and kill? It was an existential problem, one of morality-not will nor capacity. "How can I fight back at Bhisma with my arrows in battle or at Drona, Madhusudana? Both deserve my homage, enemy-slayer." (*Gita* 2, 4)

Arjuna is overwhelmed by guilt. To kill his elders and teachers is to defile and negate the nourishing sustenance he gained from them. It is to kill a part of his "self". Conflicted and compromised, his cognition and judgment impaired, and his will to act paralyzed, Arjuna formally asks for Krishna's help:

> "My nature afflicted with the vice of despair, my mind confused over what is the law, I ask what is better? Pray tell me for sure. Pray guide me, your student who asks for your help! (*Gita* 2, 7)

KRISHNA BECOMES ARJUNA'S THERAPIST

The second chapter begins with Sanjaya's description of Arjuna's despondency and Krishna's initial response to his condition:

> "Why has this mood come over to you at this bad time Arjuna, this cowardice unseemly to the noble, not leading to heaven, dishonorable? Do not act like a eunuch, Partha. It does not become you. Rid yourself of this vulgar weakness of heart, stand up, enemy-burner!" (*Gita*, 2, 2-3)

The relation between Krishna and Arjuna here is not psychotherapeutic. Krishna is acting as any warrior's exhortative charioteer would do at a time of battle and crisis. Arjuna is not moved by Krishna's rhetoric. Appeals to his

Kshatriya (warrior) duties and heavenly rewards fail to motivate him. His crisis runs deeper. He is not a warrior with cold feet shying away from battle.

Arjuna asking for Krishna's help marks the beginning of a new object relation—a psychotherapeutic relationship. It begins with a resistance and an implicit negative transference that Krishna cannot help. In the verses immediately following his plea for help, Arjuna states:

> "There is nothing I see that might dispel this sorrow that desiccates my senses. If on earth I were to obtain without rivals a kingdom, Nay even the reign of the Gods!" (*Gita*, 2, 8–9)

Arjuna is not seeking insight or understanding. He wants Krishna's approval not to fight. He is asking Krishna to justify his position. This is analogous to an analysand coming to an analyst for help and saying, "I can't do what you ask of me" and "I am not sure you can help me anyway". Arjuna is a skeptical analysand. Krishna is aware of this and proceeds accordingly. The *Gita* depicts Krishna's elegant handling of the initial negative transference.

> "*Sanjaya said:* Having spoken thus to Hrsikesa, enemy burner Gudakesa said to Govinda, 'I will not fight' and fell silent. And with a smile Hrsikesa spoke to him who sat forlorn between the two armies. The Lord said: 'You sorrow over men you should not be sorry for, and yet you speak to sage issues. The wise are not sorry for either the living or the dead.' " (*Gita*, 2, 10–11)

Krishna's smile signifies Krishna's understanding of Arjuna's resistance and his intellectualizations. Krishna's smile is striking. It is not an appropriate analytic response and suggests a patronizing attitude. However, the smile is an expression of empathy and love for the subject, analogous to a parent's response to a child whose speech is incongruent with his emotional state. Krishna's smile highlights the initial object relation-that between a child and a parent. It is not a coincidence nor a dramatic interlude that Krishna's counsel to Arjuna begins with a smile. It is an expression of Krishna's understanding of the initial transference. By smiling, Krishna is accepting both the felt and the repudiated state of Arjuna's psychic experience. Krishna's smile conveys that he knows what Arjuna is feeling and what Arjuna is capable of feeling.

CHAPTER 11: VISWARUPADARSANAM

Chapter 11 is entitled "*Viswarupadarsanam*". *Darsana* is a Sanskrit word meaning vision and sight, derived from the Sanskrit root *drs,* which means to see and comprehend. *Darsana* refers to viewing God, in whatever form but carries the very profound connotation that it is not only seeing a form of god, but actually being in his presence. "Viswa" means cosmos, and "rupa" means form. Hence, "*Viswarupadarsanam*": manifestation of the cosmic form.

Chapter 11 begins with Arjuna asking directly and brazenly to see Krishna's supreme form.

> "Now I wish to set eye on your real, supernal form, just as you have described yourself, sovereign lord, supreme person!" (Gita 11, 3)

The following verse has Arjuna toning down the directness of his request. With more humility and perhaps a preconscious intuition of Krishna's identity, Arjuna qualifies his request by adding in the next verse, "If you think that I shall be able to look upon it, lord, master of Yoga." (*Gita*, 11, 4)

Krishna answers:

> "But you shall not be able to look upon me with just your ordinary eyes. I shall give you divine sight: behold my sovereign Yoga!" (*Gita*, 11–80)

What follows is a secondary description by Sanjaya to the blind king Dhrtarastra of what Arjuna saw. What indeed Arjuna directly saw exceeds human comprehension and is beyond words. Sanjaya describes the vision as: "If in the sky the light of a thousand suns were to rise at once, it would be the likeness of the light of the great spirited one." (*Gita* 11, 9–12)

Upon seeing Krishna in his divine form, Arjuna is overwhelmed by awe and fear. His ego boundaries are distorted and obliterated. He remembers how he treated Krishna as his friend, soul mate, and his equal. Overwhelmed, ashamed, frightened and humbled in the presence of God, Arjuna asks Krishna to return to his original human form:

> "If, thinking you friend, I have too boldly cried, 'Yadava! Krishna! Come here my friend'. Not knowing of this your magnificence, out of absence of mind or sheer affection....Therefore I bow low, prostrating my body and ask for forgiveness, worshipful lord! Pray bear with me, God, as a father with son....I wish to see you again as before." (*Gita* 11, 41–46)

Arjuna's response to Krishna's divinity is fear. Note the terms Sanjaya uses to describe Arjuna's reaction: amazement, reverence, fright, thrill, fear and trembling. Perhaps the most compelling and encompassing description of the complex of emotions experienced by Arjuna is *awe*, verbatim defined in the Oxford English Dictionary (1971) as: "Immediate and active fear, terror and dread. From its use in reference to the Divine Being this passes into: Dread mingled with veneration, reverential or respectful fear; the attitude of a mind subdues to profound reverence in the presence of supreme authority, moral greatness or sublimity, or mysterious sacredness". Accordingly, Keltner and Hait (2003) note: "Awe figures prominently in religious discussions of the relationship between humans and their gods. One of the earliest and most powerful examples is found in the dramatic climax of the *Bhagavadgita*". (p. 298)

In psychoanalytic literature, Phyllis Greenacre (1956) wrote that awe derives from the phallic stage of psychosexual development, specifically, awe of the father's phallus. She notes: "One of the most interesting parts of the awe reaction is with its association with inspiration, with creativity and with *religious feelings*" (Greenacre, p. 30, italics mine). Mortimer Ostow elaborates on the role of awe in religious experience. Distinguishing fearful awe from pleasant awe, Ostow proposes, like Greenacre, that the feeling of awe experienced by adults has its origins in the infant's preverbal sensory experience of his parents, and writes, more persuasively than Greenacre, that "The sense of awe derives from the newborn's nondeclarative memory of his impressions of his adult, giant parents." (Ostow, p. 231) Ostow correctly emphasizes the visual perception of disproportionate scales of size as central to the feeling of awe. Dwarkanath Rao, in his paper, "God Playing Psychoanalyst: Lessons From the Bhagavad Gita" arrives at the same point, stating: "One wonders if the cosmic vision of Krishna can be understood as the terrifying, omnipotent, omniscient parent of vulnerable childhood." (Rao, p. 183)

Keltner and Hait discuss the cognitive development of awe as relating to importance of size and scale from within the Piagetian framework of accommodation. They write:

> "Accommodation refers to the Piagetian process of adjusting mental structures that cannot assimilate a new experience. The concept of accommodation brings together many insights about awe, such as that it involves confusion (St. Paul) and obscurity (Burke), and that is heightened in times of crisis, when extant traditions and knowledge structures do not suffice (Weber). We propose that prototypical awe involves a challenge to or negation of mental structures when they fail to make sense of an experience of something vast. Such experiences can be disorienting and even frightening, as in the cases of Arjuna and St. Paul, since they make the self-feel small, powerless, and confused."(p. 304)

The cognitive understanding of awe reinforces the importance psychoanalysts place on the interpersonal and emotional dimensions of awe: both describe the early developmental experiences of a child trying to comprehend and assimilate an experience that is beyond their cognitive and maturational ability.

THE VISUAL REALM: SEEING IS BELIEVING

Most of the *Gita* occurs within the realm of speech. Krishna talks, and Arjuna listens and questions. Chapter 11 is the notable exception, wherein vision and sight figure predominantly. Indeed, Krishna gives Arjuna divine vision to view his cosmic self: *"I give you divine sight".* The role of vision and sight are critical to Arjuna's spiritual conversion, as it is through the eyes that Arjuna takes in Krishna and identifies with his divinity. It is through seeing that Arjuna understands what Krishna tells him in chapter 10: "Of the Sons of Pandu, I am Arjuna".

In psychoanalytic theory, seeing is often intimately associated with internalizations: with eating and devouring. Literally, "eating with one's eyes." Going back to chapter 11 of the *Gita,* Arjuna, having seen Krishna's divine form, says: "You are greedily licking your lips to devour these worlds entire with your flickering mouths" (Gita, 11: 29). Note the explicit imagery of devouring. On the surface level, it implies destruction. On a psychoanalytic level, it is also a mechanism of identification with the *other*. The equation would be: looking = devouring = oral incorporation = introjection = identification. In Otto Fenichel's words:

> "Whenever conformity to the demands of another person involves *looking up* to him we have, on the one hand, a proof of the existence of ocular introjection... There are hundreds of different instances of this sort. For example, he who stumbles looks at the image of God and stands firm again. Or, we derive moral strength by looking at the picture of someone whom we desire to copy—the very word 'copy' implies looking... it is not merely a question of reinforcing one's moral courage by acquiring visual evidence that other people are moral and that they behave in such and such a way. Rather it is a question of *the magical properly of a look*: through the look itself the characteristics of that which is looked at are acquired by the person who looks." (Fenichel, 1937)

Witness the "magical" properties of looking that Fenichel stresses: by "looking", one is mysteriously, even miraculously taking in the "other". For Arjuna, looking at Krishna's cosmic self-amounts to an identification with God. Arjuna's mundane consciousness is converted to a higher spiritual level through the act of looking—no ordinary looking, and no ordinary identification. It is looking at God himself and identifying with him. Such identification may appear presumptuous and narcissistic, but it is in keeping with the Hindu philosophical paradigm that the spiritual unconditioned "self" is present, though hidden and obfuscated, in all of us by the bodily conditioned, mundane self.

The role of vision (of ocular introjection as mechanism of identification in Arjuna's conversion) is highly relevant to the Hindu practice of worship. The climax in the Hindu ritual of worship is to view the Deity. This is called a "*darshan*". The notion of seeing, as a *darshan,* has an important place in Hindu ritual worship. It underlies the basis for the more gradual approach for the everyday man to approach God and spiritual understanding. A *darshan* is not a unique or singular event, as was Krishna's theophany, but the norm of everyday practice of Hinduism. After the priest makes oblations to the God, the devotees place their hands in reverence as they view the deity in the inner sanctorum. The viewing of the Deity, the *darshan*, can be emotionally translated as being in presence of God. The stone or bronze deity in a typical temple takes on a magical significance of *being God.* This is not a mental nor a physical representation. It is considered a concrete and actual presence. However, the emotion is short lived. Just as Arjuna's vision of the divine was brief—he in fact begged for it to end-so too is the *darshan*. The feeling of being present in, with, and within God—a power far greater than oneself—both nullifies and edifies the ego, negating the mundane self and edifying the transcendent self. Being, however transiently, in the presence of God, seeing, experiencing and taking him in, makes one more receptive to similar states. It motivates and permits one to a more permanent, internalized relationship with the Deity.

In the novel *Anil's Ghost*, Michael Ondaatje, a noted Sri Lankan author, writes about artisans painting images of the divine Buddha. It was considered heresy to paint the eyes directly. This would mean looking into the deities' eyes as they were created: an act of reverence but also of fear, trepidation and retribution through the human encountering the divine, with all its Oedipal connotations. Thus, when artisans created painted deities, they could only paint the eyes by looking at their work through a mirror.

> Without the eyes there is not just blindness, there is nothing. There is no existence. The artificer brings to life sight and truth and presence... He climbs a ladder in front of the statue. The man with him climbs too. This has taken place for centuries, you realize, there are records of this since the ninth century. The painter dips a brush into the paint and turns back to the statue, so it looks as if it is to be enfolded in the great arms. The other man, facing him, holds up the mirror, and the artificer puts the brush over his shoulder and paints in the eyes without looking directly at the face. He uses just the reflection to guide him—so only the mirror receives the direct image of the glance being created. No human eye can meet the Buddha's during the process of creation...he never looks at the eyes directly. He can only see the gaze in the mirror. (Ondaatje 2000: 99)

The relation between Krishna and Arjuna continues as analyst and analysand, but another parallel object-relation develops in and after chapter 11 that between devotee (*Bhakta*) and God. Krishna says to Arjuna:

> "You have seen this rarely revealed form that is mine. Even the gods always yearn for a glimpse of this form. Thus, as I am and as you have seen me, I cannot be seen with the aid of the Vedas, austerities, gifts and sacrifices. Only through exclusive *Bhakti* can I be seen thus, Arjuna, and known as I really am, and entered into. Only he comes to me, Pandava,

who acts for me, who holds me as the highest, who is devoted to me without self-interest, and without any animosity against any creature." (*Gita* 11, 52–55)

This is *Bhakti* defined by the God Krishna himself. *Bhakti* means devotion or "love of god". It is not an intellectual love but an intense emotional and affective experience. *Bhakti* is a personal relation between the individual and God, without the middleman, the priest. A necessary condition for *Bhakti* is surrender to the object of *Bhakti*. The ego suspends itself to a state where it becomes selfless and egoless. In other words, self-love (narcissism) is directed towards object love. In drive theory, narcissistic libido becomes invested in object libido, the object being God. Freud noted that such a condition occurs in only one instance—the state of being in love.

From a psychoanalytic stance, *Bhakti* and the religious sentiments accompanying it are often seen as defenses against infantile dependence and narcissistic regression to a primordial blissful dyadic infant-mother state. Such a reductionistic view does not allow for the possibility of a developmentally advanced and healthy sources of faith and religious belief. Compare Freud's notion of "*thanatos*" or the death instinct to Krishna's description of who he is: "I am time grown old". Sandor Ferenczi, in his work *Thalassa*, considers Freud's concept of the death instinct and regression to symbiotic union with the mother in a manner that more closely approximates the Hindu essence. Ferenczi writes:

> "There does not exist an absolute life without any admixture of symptoms of death, biology has long asserted; and it is but a short while since that that Freud demonstrated the operation of the death instinct among all living things. 'The goal of all life is death', for 'lifelessness was here before life was'. What if. however, death and dying were not anything absolute, if germs of life and regressive tendencies lay hidden even within inorganic matter. If Nietzsche were right when he said, 'All inorganic matter has originated out of the organic, it is dead organic matter. Corpse and man.' Then we should have to drop once and for all the question of the beginning and end of life, and conceive the whole inorganic and organic world as a perpetual oscillating between the will to live and the will to die in which an absolute hegemony on part either of life or of death is never attained." (Ferenczi, 1938, p. 94–95)

CONCLUSION

I have approached the *Bhagavad Gita* as a psychological discourse. The interaction between Arjuna and Krishna can be viewed as a psychotherapeutic process, replete with resistances, transferences and cognitive distortions.

I have assiduously not dealt with the subject matter of the *Gita*, because the *Gita* as a religious text contains assumptions that psychoanalysis does not admit.

Arjuna's crisis is precipitated by the Oedipal guilt of killing paternal surrogates. The sensory modality of vision—actually seeing God—is central to Arjuna's conversion and his subsequent identification with God. The overwhelming feelings of awe, wonder and fear of seeing Krishna as God figure importantly in the change and alteration in Arjuna's consciousness and his spiritual conversion. The overwhelming scale of the divine vision is necessary to jolt Arjuna's ordinary consciousness to a higher spiritual level, providing an ideal greater in magnitude and intensity to his guilt. The spiritual conversion that is affected by seeing God as a frightening and incomprehensible entity has its psychological antecedents in the infant's perception of his parents as powerful and fearful and yet loving and caring. The worship of an all-powerful Divinity dissolves and absolves the child in us of our inevitable patricidal guilt, as embodied by Arjuna, Avatar for us all.

NOTE

All references to the *Bhagavad Gita* are from JAB van Buitenen's translation. References to the *Gita* are in the form of chapter, followed by the verse. For example, *Gita,* 2:1-3 means chapter 2, verses 1-3. This allows the reader to readily cross reference the citation to any one of the multiple translations of the *Gita* that are available.

FURTHER READING

1. Abraham K. "The Influence of Oral Eroticism on Character Formation". In Selected Papers of Karl Abrahan. New York, Brunner/Mazel. 1924. pp. 393-406.
2. Ferenczi S. Thalassa: A Theory of Genitality. New York: Norton & Company; 1938.
3. Freud A. The Ego and the Mechanisms of Defense. New York: International Universities Press; 1966.
4. Freud S. "An outline of psychoanalysis." Standard edition. 1940;23:143-207.
5. Greenacre P. "Experiences of awe in childhood." Psychoanalytic Study of the Child. 1956;11: 9-30.
6. James W. "The Varieties of Religious Experience", Penguin Classics; 1985.
7. Karve I. "Yuganta: The End of an Epoch." Hyderabad, India: Disha Books; 1991.
8. Loewald H. "On the Therapeutic Action of Psychoanalysis." Int J Psychoanal. 1960;41:16-33.
9. Mahler MS, Pine F, Bergman A. The Psychological Birth of the Human Infant. New York: Basic Books; 1975.
10. Ostow M. "Three archaic contributions to the religious instinct: awe, mysticism, and apocalypse." In: Akhtar S, Parens H (Eds). Does God Help?: Developmental, Psychological, and Technical Aspects of Religious Belief. Northvale, NJ: Jason Aronson; 2001.

11. Oxford English Dictionary. Oxford, England: Oxford University Press; 1971.
12. Rao DG. "God playing psychoanalyst". In: Akhtar S, Parens H. Does God Help?: Developmental, Psychological, and Technical Aspects of Religious Belief. Northvale, NJ: Jason Aronson; 2001.
13. The Mahabharata. Trans. Dutt, MN. Delhi, India: Parimal; 1994.
14. Van Buitenen JAB. The Bhagavad Gita in the Mahabharata. Chicago: University of Chicago Press; 1980.
15. Winnicott D, (1960). "Theory of the Parent-Infant Relationship". Int J Psychoanal. 1960;40:585-95.

8 CHAPTER Yoga and Mindfulness-based Cognitive Therapy (Y-MBCT)

Basant Pradhan

"Yoga is nothing but harnessing the mind to unharness itself of the memories and desires"

—**Wilfred Bion: *Psychoanalytic Forum* (1967)**

ABSTRACT

Yoga is nothing but practical psychology and meditation is not an action: rather, it is a state of mind in which there exists concurrently alertness, relaxation and responsiveness, not reactivity. These are states of *being* rather than doing. Meditation is part of Yoga, and mindfulness is one of the two types of meditation. To be specific, in the ancient Indian spiritual traditions, the 6th and 7th limbs of the *eight-limbed Yoga* are widely regarded as the corpus of meditation. Despite their prevailing history from millennia, their profound philosophies and ever-increasing scopes and utilities, many aspects of Yoga and meditation are still quite misunderstood, more so in the Western world. The many distorted views surrounding Yoga and meditation adds further to the lack of clarity as to what they mean in practice, especially in clinical settings, thus posing as the major hurdles for their effective integration into healthcare. Furthermore, the development of disorder specific Yoga- and meditation-based treatment models and their targeted uses are rather lacking although there is burgeoning of the fragmented or piecemeal use of Yoga and meditation, mainly for weight loss or stress reduction, etc., usages far from their original propositions. This is in sharp contrast to the original propositions in the ancient India in which Yoga was viewed as an all-encompassing *eight-stepped process*, e.g., sage Patanjali's *Eight-limbed Yoga* or the Buddha's *Noble Eight-fold Path*. The Yoga and mindfulness-based cognitive therapy (Y-MBCT) modules are fusion models which are Pradhan's humble attempts to bridge some of the existing treatment gaps in many neuropsychiatric conditions. Embarking upon these aspects and drawing from the original traditions, this chapter provides information on the various ways to attain the mindfulness states and to apply these enhanced mental states in user-friendly and evidence-based ways to enhance our health and wellbeing.

Keywords: Yoga, Meditation, Mindfulness, Psychotherapy, Cognitive behavioral therapy (CBT)

THE COGNITIVE PSYCHOLOGY OF YOGA AND ITS EXTENSION FOR PSYCHOTHERAPY: ANCIENT INDIAN PERSPECTIVES

The Psychology of Yoga

Aurobindo, a philosopher and mystic of the pre-independent India (20th century), informs us that "*Yoga is nothing but practical psychology*"

(Aurobindo, 1999). *Psychology* is the systematic study of the mind, the spectrum of the various mental states and the ensuing experiences co-constructed by the various mental phenomena (Pali. *dhama*). *Psychotherapy* ('talk therapy') is the clinically applied aspect of psychology that eventually facilitates one's progress towards wellbeing and finding the meaning and purpose in one's life. A central goal of Yoga is to *know thyself:* to find the deep meanings of one's life so that one can attain self-actualization. Psychology of Yoga is essentially humanistic. Yogic psychology claims that the basic ingredients of happiness are present inside everybody and happiness can be cultivated in a systematic manner by embracing its philosophies, techniques and praxes, i.e., the *trilogy* of Yoga. Yoga is a self-care, a home coming. From time immemorial, Yoga and meditation have been conceptualized as self-management strategies for gaining deep knowledge (insight; Pali. *nana*) into the structural constituents (Sanskrit. *chitta*) and operating principles or doctrines (Pali. *dhama*) of the human mind that explain the *true* nature of our thoughts and experiences. Mind always plays tricks with us: These insights help us to experience calmness in sustained manner *regardless of the circumstances of our daily life,* enables us to reaccess the natural and positive states of the mind, and how to use these enhanced states of the mind for our wellbeing. In that sense, Yoga is a *positive psychology* (Seligman and Csikszentmihalyi, 2000). The deep wisdom of the Yogic philosophies informs us that our *inside* (i.e., the mind) is the seat of all our experiences. Thus, self-realization (to *know thyself*), i.e., application of a series of *introjections* into one's life can occur *only from the within,* by developing inner self-knowledge (*insight*; Sanskrit. *jnana*). This cannot be attained by merely focusing on the external world, by sole use of *projective* mechanisms. Rather, one needs to have introspective self-analysis in nonjudgmental manner, that is meditation, the science of inner engineering. This helps to develop further one's inside (i.e., the mind): in the *Abhidhammic* psychology (Buddhist Pali canon), this is called *moral development,* an integral part of meditative life (Ingram, 2008). In other words, *moral development* by use of meditation can *upgrade* one's mind to higher grades so that one's *views* (Sanskrit. *drishti*) on life become purified. Yoga as an elaborate system with its rich philosophies, elaborate techniques and systematized praxes provides us with the science and technology necessary to study and regulate the mind and remediate its pathologies so that self-actualization becomes attainable.

Codification of Yoga and Meditation in the Eight-stepped Methods

As the early *compilers* (not inventors) of Yoga and meditation in the ancient India, the major contributions of the Buddha (circa 6th century BC) and sage teacher Patanjali (circa. 400 BC) were proposition of the *eight-stepped methods*, i.e., Buddha's Noble Eight-fold Path (Pali. *Atthangika Magga*, Bodhi, 2000; Nanamoli, 1956; Gunaratana, 2009) and Patanjali's Eight-limbed Yoga (Sanskrit. *ashtanga*; Satchidananda, 1978) in which meditation was part of Yoga. Buddha's extraordinary contribution was specifically on meditation, especially its systematization and further development within the broader system of Yoga. Building further upon the existing meditative methods, he developed the *mindfulness type of meditation* (Pali. *satipatthana* method: Nanamoli, 1995), as a solution to the myriads of problems presented to us by the mind and life. Radically departing from the contemporary ascetic traditions which included many extreme practices, Buddha proposed the *Middle Way*: the path of moderation rather than extremism (Dalai Lama, 2009). The Middle Way, due to its simplicity, ease and pragmatism, enabled the ordinary people of ancient India to be meditators while living in their households: they did not need to go the hermitages in the forests: it paved the way for meditation to be a way of life for the common mass. The Noble Eightfold Path, with mindfulness embedded in it, was the prescription of the Buddha for transcending the human sufferings. No wonder, the *Abhidhammic* scriptures (Pali canon) described Buddha as a physician of his time. Studying the Buddha's own life, one realizes that based on his personal experience of the sudden and severe sufferings he was exposed to, he experimented with the utility of mindfulness for himself (for 7-year) and ended his own sufferings by achieving enlightenment (Santina, 1997). After successful application of mindfulness on himself, he proposed it as a solution for the amelioration of the sufferings of all sentient beings. As elaborated in the *Abhidhammic* texts (Pali canon), Buddha had abandoned many aspects of the Vedic doctrines such as cosmology and metaphysical aspects and focused instead on their experiential and pragmatic aspects. As Eliade (1958) points out elegantly, "Buddha always closely connected knowledge with a meditational experience of the Yogic type. For him knowledge was of little value so long as it was not *realized* in the personal experience of it." To him, all the truths must be tested in Yogic fashion—that is, must be meditated and experienced. To Buddha, the direct experience meditation, as realized through the moments at hand, was of primary importance: he chose 'experience' over 'knowledge', for him, the former had the primacy. That is *the true spirit* for the use of meditation for psychotherapy and wellbeing. Approaching psychotherapy in this way, the guidance comes from the insights gained from our lived experiences, not just from the book knowledge.

Yoga and Psychotherapy

The *Bhagavad Gita* (Holy scripture of the Hindu traditions; Yogananda, 1995) claims that the root of all suffering is the agitation or endless fluctuation of the mind, the consequence of selfish desire (Sanskrit. *kamana*; Pali. *tanha*).

A powerful method to extinguish this desire is by steadying and pacifying the mind through the path of meditation. This allows the practitioner (*Yogi*) to gain self-knowledge (Pali. *nana*) or insight (Pali. *vipassana*) and move up in the spiritual path to eventually attain liberation (Sanskrit. *moksha*) from the sufferings. This reminds us of Bion's (British psychoanalytic thinker) description of Yoga as *harnessing the mind to unharness itself of memory and desire* (Bion 1967). Simiar to Patanjali's description on Yoga (circa. 400 BC), Bion suggested that desire and memory are the enemies of the attention in the psychoanalytic processes. Buddha in his various discourses (Pali. *nikaya*) on meditation, and the sage teacher Patanjali in the *Yoga Sutras,* attest that the main process in deep meditative states (Sanskrit. *samadhis;* Pali. *samapattis*) involves maintaining a *dispassionate attitude to make oneself free of the desires* as well as getting past one's *engraved mental impressions* (deep memories, Sanskrit. *samskaras*). The Buddha has labeled this dispassionate attitude as the *non-clinging* stance. One can note here a technical similarity between Yoga and psychoanalysis: a dispassionate or detached exploration of these engraved memories in Yoga vs. the psychoanalytic method to recollect, reconstitute and assimilate one's memories of early childhood (Eliade, 1969). The goal is same, i.e., to obtain a corrected understanding (insight).

Yoga, as proposed originally, was inclusive of meditation, and was conceptualized as a process of introspective self-analysis that involves nonjudgmental investigations and reappraisals of the various internal states using that very mind as the instrument to study these mental states (Pradhan, 2014). Yoga proposes to use the reflexive powers of the mind in looking back into its own depths, with a broader goal of transcending the sufferings of mankind through liberation from the constraints of the mind. Psychotherapy, as proposed by Freud (1915), uses the same power of mind to resolve its basic conflicts. Yoga has also been defined as the method of unifying the *lower* or egoistic mind (Sanskrit. *manasa*) to the *higher* mind (Sanskrit. *buddhi,* the discriminative faculty of mind) through meditation (Feuerstein 1990). Thus, one can see that Yogic philosophies do propose a hierarchical or graded system of mind, from lower to higher to the highest, in some ways similar to Freud's propositions, e.g., the topographical—(*preconscious, conscious,* and *unconscious*) and structural—(*id, ego,* and *superego*) models of the mind (Freud, 1915). In the existential sense, Yoga is the science of self-realization. The goal of Yoga is to transcend the sufferings of life, to find the deep meanings of one's life so that one can attain self-actualization, a major goal of the *positive psychology* (Seligman and Csikszentmihalyi, 2000). Yoga has been a way of life for the common mass of India from ancient times so much so that it will not be an exaggeration to say that history of Yoga is that of India itself for the most part. The entire system of the *Ayurveda* (ancient Indian system of healing) has been based on the Yogic philosophies (Frawley, 1999). Self-analysis is a goal common to both Yoga as well as any analytically-oriented psychotherapy (such as psychoanalysis). Both Yoga and psychotherapy are investigative and analytic pursuits to understand the intricate nature of the human mind, the methods in both are drawn from universally applicable theories of the mind and, obtaining the self-knowledge or insight (Sanskrit. *jnana*; Pali. *nana, vipassana*) is the foundational tenet in both for amelioration of the human sufferings. Thus, Yoga and psychotherapy have many things in common, including some common goals. Contemporary Indian psychiatry also considers spirituality as a core ingredient of mental health. *Bhagavad Gita,* or *Song of the Lord* (Yogananda, 1995), is a Hindu philosophical scripture that exemplifies the principles of psychotherapy, especially insight-oriented, client-centered, motivational, behavioral, and existential. Written by Sage Vyasa (c. 4–5 BCE) in the form of a dialogue between the battle-conflicted and despondent prince Arjuna (the client) and his charioteer Lord Krishna (the psychotherapist) in the epic *Mahabharata* (similar to Homer's Iliad and Odyssey). In this epic consisting of over 700 verses, the dialogue on Yoga and meditation occurs in its 2nd chapter ("Sankhya and Yoga") and 6th chapter ("Permanent Shelter in Spirit through Yoga and Meditation") as well. Psychotherapy in India often incorporates therapeutic pearls from the Bhagavad Gita (Venkoba Rao, 1978; Reddy, 2012). From time immemorial, *Yoga has been the psychotherapy of the East.*

YOGA INCLUDES MEDITATION AS ITS 6TH AND 7TH STEPS: THE EIGHT-STEPPED METHODS OF THE BUDDHA AND PATANJALI

Misconceptions Surrounding Yoga and Meditation

Despite their prevailing history from millennia, their profound philosophies and ever-increasing scopes and utilities, many aspects of Yoga and meditation are still quite misunderstood, more so in the Western world. The myriads of unauthentic ways they are being practiced in today's modern world are quite discordant and divergent from the original propositions and prescriptions: thus, perpetuating further the misconceptions and mysteries surrounding these powerful practices. In the West, Yoga is largely (mis-) understood as a physical exercise or a postural technique, and meditation as a breathing technique: quite a dichotomous view. The many distorted views surrounding Yoga and meditation adds further to the lack of clarity as to what they mean in practice, especially in clinical settings, thus posing as the major hurdles for their effective integration into healthcare. Furthermore, the development of disorder specific Yoga- and meditation-based treatment models and their targeted use are rather lacking although there is burgeoning of the fragmented or piecemeal use of Yoga and meditation, mainly for weight loss or stress reduction, etc., usages far from their original propositions. Sadly, in these unintegrated and distorted formats, one finds that the physical aspects of Yoga are over-emphasized and the philosophical and the psychological aspects are rather neglected.

The Eight-stepped Methods of the Buddha and Patanjali: An Illustrated Summary

This dichotomous and distorted view of Yoga and meditation is in sharp contrast to the original propositions in the spiritual traditions of the ancient India in which Yoga was viewed as all-encompassing *eight-stepped methods.* These are *Patanjali's Eight-limbed Yoga* (Sanskrit. *ashtanga;* Satchidananda, 1978) or the Buddha's *Noble Eight-fold Path* (Pali. *Atthangika Magga*, Bodhi, 2000; Nanamoli, 1956): the propositions for *use of Yoga in its entirety* (all eight steps) rather than piecemeal. In them, meditation was an integral part of Yoga, the higher meditative states are the culmination points in Yoga. To be specific, the 6th and 7th limbs of the *eight-limbed Yoga* were widely regarded as the corpus of meditation proper (Taimni, 1961). These 6th and 7th limbed are popularly known as *concentration* (attention; Sanskrit. *dharana*) and mindfulness (detached awareness; Sanskrit. *dhyana*) respectively (Satchidananda, 1978; Nyanaponika, 1954). In these original propositions, mindfulness (Pali. *satipatthana*) was regarded as one of the two types of meditation, the other type being known as concentration (Pali. *samatha*) (Analayo, 2003). *Concentration* is derived from a Sanskrit word *dharana,* which literally means an 'attentional anchor' to tether the wandering mind. Thus, it is no surprise that concentration practice is often considered as a prerequisite before one is able to attain the mindful state (Ingram, 2008; Pradhan, 2014). As Feuerstein (2001) explains: "Yoga provides us with inner stability and balance, both of which depend upon constant concentration."

As demonstrated in **Figure 1**, the *eight-stepped methods* include the Yogic life-style (*Buddha's Middle Way*, elaborated later), preparation of the body and aligning the various parts of the mind (*the five-factors of the mind,* elaborated later) which eventually leads to the deep meditative states (*samadhi*), the culmination of Yoga. These eight-stepped methods can be summed up into three categories (Ingram, 2008; Dalai Lama, 2009):

1. Meditative life-style (*the Middle Way, the path of moderation*): *Steps 1 and 2.*
2. Preparations for- and practice of concentration (Pali. samatha): *Steps 3 to 6.*
3. Practice of *mindfulness* (Pali. *vipassana*): *Step 7.* Buddha's *satipatthana* is the systematized method to practice *vipassana* which gives rise to *insight/ wisdom* (Sanskrit. *jnana*). The *wisdom* eventually results in the *liberation* (the *step 8,* Sanskrit. *moksha*) from the sufferings.

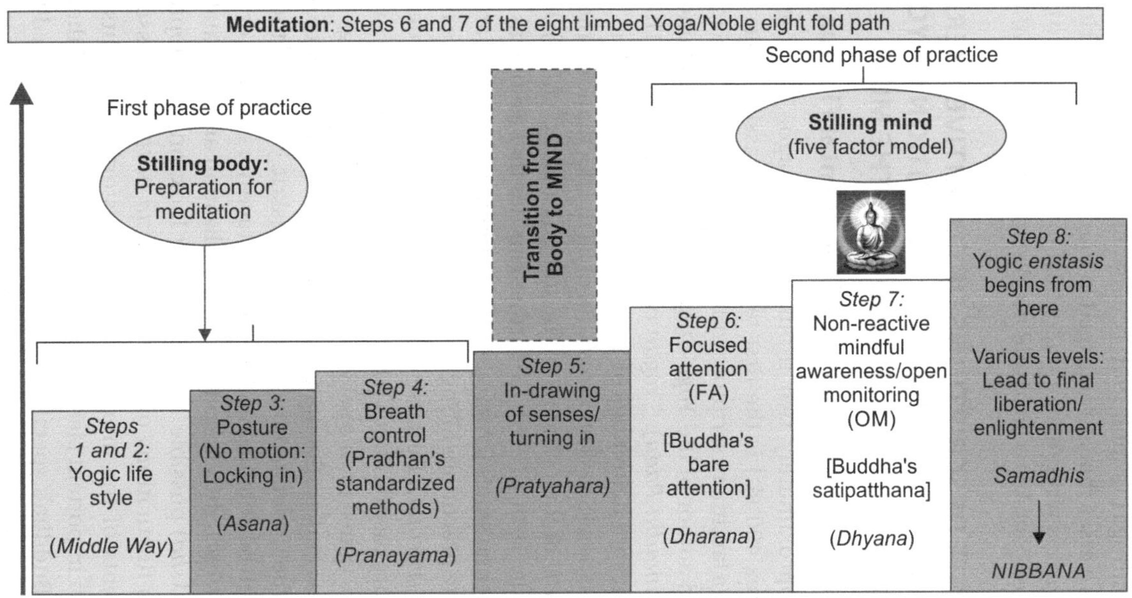

Fig. 1: The *eight-stepped methods* in yoga and meditation.

For any meditation training and practice to be successfully used in one's daily life situations, these *three aspects* need to be practiced in the eight sequential steps, as illustrated above. Elaborate descriptions of the *Eight-limbed Yoga* can be found in *Patanjali's Yoga-Sutra,* the first textbook on Yoga (Taimni, 1961; Feuerstein, 1979). Consisting of 196 terse aphorisms/verses that are arranged in four sections (Sanskrit. *pada*), the *Yoga-Sutra* was written as a dialectical form (conversation) between a Yoga Master (Sanskrit. *Guru*) and the disciples (Sanskrit. *sadhaka*).

ELABORATE DESCRIPTIONS OF COGNITIVE THERAPY ARE FOUND IN PATANJALI'S EARLY DEFINITION OF YOGA AND BUDDHA'S FIVE-FACTOR MODEL OF THE MIND

Yoga Defined as the Cessation of the Mental Fluctuations

Compiled approximately two thousand years ago, *The Yoga-Sutra of Patanjali* (circa 400 BC) is the first textbook on classical Yoga (*the Eight-limbed Yoga*): a landmark scripture indeed (Feuerstein, 1979). Sage Patanjali, the celebrated author of the *Yoga-Sutra,* defines Yoga in its famous verse-2 (Section-I, *Samadhi Pada*): "*Yogah chitta vritti nirodhah.*" This is one of the most significant definitions of Yoga and literally means that "Yoga is the control or cessation (Sanskrit: *nirodhah*) of all the fluctuations/modifications (Sanskrit: *vritti)* of the contents of the mind (Sanskrit: *chitta*) at all levels" (Satchidananda, 1978, p. 3–6). He further clarifies that as long as these ever-fluctuating mental states (*chitta-vrittis)* are not in a state of balance or poise (*nirodhah*), the practitioner (Yogi) is not established in his true nature (true self; Sanskrit. *svarupa*). Because of these fluctuations, he misidentifies with these temporary mental states (*chitta-vrittis*) and his views become afflicted by the *illusions* (Sanskrit. *maya*) which begets him the sufferings of life. Only by ceasing these endless fluctuations of mind through the practice of Yoga and meditation, true understandings (insight, Sanskrit. *jnana*) of these endless fluctuations can be obtained and we can embrace our essential or *true* nature (Sanskrit: *svarupa*), thus making the self-realization and eventual liberation (Sanskrit: *moksha*) possible. Taking a closer look, one can appreciate that these endless fluctuations of the mind (*chitta-vrittis)* are essentially the various contents of the mind such as the distorted thoughts (*cognitive distortions*), an important element of the cognitive behavioral therapy (CBT; Beck, 1976). Buddha's specific contribution to Yoga and meditation was further development of the path of meditation (Pali. *satipatthana* method) using the broader framework of Yoga—a corpus of Yogic knowledge burrowed from his earlier teachers such as Alara Kalama and Uddaka Ramaputta of the *Indus Valley civilization* traditions (Eliade, 1958; Santina, 1997). Buddha's proposition was that the central goal of meditation is to facilitate the union of the liberating cognitions (Pali. *nanas*) and the insight (Pali. *vipassana*), both of which emanate from the meditative process so that one can obtain liberation from the sufferings inherent to the human condition (Ingram, 2008). For these liberating cognitions and insights to ensue from the meditative process and for their union to result in liberation from the human sufferings, the methods in the *Noble Eightfold Path* of the Buddha and the *Eight-limbed Yoga* of Patanjali serve as clear road maps for the practitioner. Here again one can appreciate the importance of the right thoughts (cognitions) and insights that result from meditation—similar to those in the cognitive behavior therapy (CBT) and psychodynamic psychotherapy respectively. It is very pertinent to describe the five-factor model of the mind that will make such similarities even clearer.

Mind as a Bundle of Five Things: Buddha's Five-factor Model

In the Yogic philosophies, the mind is conceptualized as another *internal apparatus* (Sanskrit. *antah-karana*), the sixth sense organ, similar to the other five. As initially elaborated by the Buddha in the oral tradition (circa 6th century BC) and later on canonized in the Pali texts of the *Abhidhamma,* mind is a bundle of five things, the five factors (Pradhan, 2014. pp. 42–43). The mind expresses itself through these five components which co-construct the experiences in our daily life **(Fig. 2)**.

These five components are the *thoughts, feelings, sensations/perceptions, urges/impulses* that express in behavior, and *memories*. This is the *five-factor model* of the mind, as proposed by the Buddha. Pradhan adapted this concept and developed the *five-factor inventory* of human experience, for its disorder specific therapeutic use in the chronic and difficult experiences involved in conditions such as pain, trauma, addiction or psychosis (Pradhan and Pinninti, 2016. pp.70–72; Pradhan, 2017. pp. 224–227; Pradhan, Pinninti and Rathod, 2019). Taking a closer look, one can appreciate the similarities between the *thought record* (Beck, 1976) used in the cognitive behavioral therapy (CBT) and the *five-factor inventory*. Thought record has three aspects (thoughts, feelings, and behavior) whereas the five-factor inventory has two additional aspects, i.e., sensations/perceptions and memories as well.

Let's examine further the similarities between Yogic philosophies and cognitive therapy from the perspective of *cognitive reappraisal* (Lazarus and Alfert, 1964). Cognitive reappraisal is a primary form of cognitive change which is defined as changing the way one thinks about a situation in order to change its emotional impact. It entails using cognitive and linguistic processes to reframe or reformulate the meaning of a situation in order to regulate the emotions, especially the negative ones. One sees a similar description in the Yogic philosophies from the ancient India. Yogic philosophies claim that our day to day experiences in the ordinary sense are just representations in the

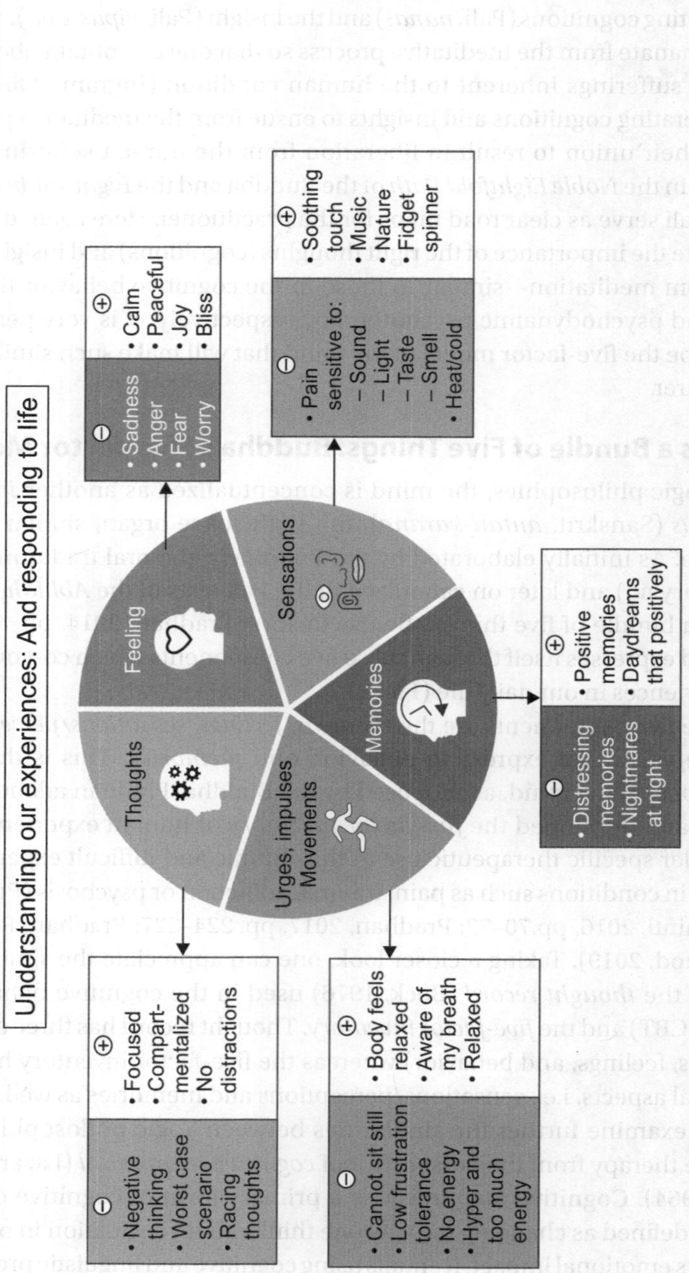

Fig. 2: The five factors of the mind that co-construct our experiences.

mind, i.e., they are symbolic rather than real (they are maps, not territories). These experiences are dependent on the grade/quality of the mind and they keep on changing with the change of the conditions of the mind that invoked such representations (simulations). Because all representations can be tricked and are changeable based on the state of the mind, the Buddha and Patanjali have advised us *not to cling* to these representations, i.e., not to consider our thoughts as real facts, rather to take them as mere thoughts and watch them from a distance. This is essentially a *cognitive reappraisal,* a central technique employed in many psychotherapies, CBT and psychodynamic psychotherapy alike. Such reappraisals using the reflective power of the mind prevents our indulgence into the thoughts and endless ruminations. As mentioned before, because of the elusive and projective properties of the sensorial mind, *our perception of reality is rather a virtual reality.* The origin of stress lies precisely here, in our very (mis-) perceptions. Problems (such as stress, psychological symptoms) arise when we mistake these representations as facts (mistaking the map as the territory) because of our rigid (mis-) identifications with these representations, thus creating an *illusion* (Sanskrit. *maya*) in the way we view our situations. Such erroneous beliefs (Sanskrit. *avidya*) make us to jump onto quick conclusions based on incomplete information. These concepts are very similar to the *cognitive distortions* described in CBT (Beck, 1976). One such cognitive distortion is the *arbitrary inference*—jumping into conclusions based on incomplete/false information. Yoga and psychotherapy, both agree that such distortions and erroneous beliefs, if not corrected with the new insights (Sanskrit. *jnana*) gained from our life experiences, do prevent us from updating these (mis-) representations in the mind and in many ways, become the sources of our sufferings. One can see here that management of our problems of daily life is actually management of our own misperceptions (distortions) by obtaining the internal knowledge about the self—the insights (Pali. *vipassana*). In that sense, Yogic philosophies are nothing but psychotherapies based on self-analysis, deep knowledge about the mind and its various modus operandi, strengths, as well as limitations and the various ways to strengthen or purify it so that our cognitive distortions and the resulting misperceptions can be corrected. Thus, the similarities between Yoga and psychotherapies such as CBT cannot be clearer.

MEDITATION AS DETACHED OBSERVATION ('CALM NOTICING'): AN ILLUSTRATED SUMMARY

Meditation, simply stated as "training of the mind," is the conscious and purposeful self-regulation of one's attention to achieve stillness/poise in one's body and mind. Meditation is not an action: rather, it is a *state of mind* in which there exists concurrently alertness, relaxation and responsiveness, not reactivity (Pradhan, 2014). These are states of *being* rather than doing. Technically meditation involves *at least three components* (Tang et al., 2015): (1) Attentional control, (2) Affect regulation, and (3) A heightened sense of perception and self-awareness—an altered consciousness. These three aspects collectively support our physical and mental health, resilience, wellbeing, and behavior change. Practice of meditation essentially begins with preparing the body for this process followed by cultivating states of stable attention so that using the attention as a raft, one can observe in a nonreactive/nonjudgmental manner the changes inside the mind—the mental flux, the constant inner chatter. As far as the use and monitoring of one's attention are concerned, *all meditations are categorized into two types*: *concentration* type (Pali. *samatha*) and, *mindfulness* type (Pali. *satipatthana*) (Lutz et al., 2008). The concentration type is otherwise called *focused attention* (FA) and the mindfulness type is called *open monitoring* (OM). Thus, in FA type, the attention is focused, narrow and exclusive whereas in OM type, the attention is wide, inclusive and uniformly hovering—suitable for creating the states of nonjudgmental *awareness*. Concentration leads to one's merger/absorption into the object of meditation (Pali. *kasina*) whereas mindfulness helps us to remain detached/neutral from our experiences and thus, lessens our reactivity—we become responsive rather than reactive.

Mind is always in an ever-changing state: Meditation induces nonreactivity of the mind so that it becomes possible to observe nonjudgmentally the ongoing stream of experiences as they arise in one's awareness. This is done by establishing a focused and flexible attention on the breath or other meditation objects (Pali. *kasina*) and creating a nonjudgmental awareness of them (Pradhan et al., 2019; Pradhan, 2014). Meditation practice allows our thoughts, feelings, or sensations just to *arise and pass away* in our field of awareness while we try to maintain a specific attentional stance. This enables us to get clear glimpses of the doings of the mind: it eventually leads to a state of *detached observation* of our mental contents, i.e., the five factors of the mind. This detached observation is the process of stepping outside the mind (the five components) so that we can observe the mind from a distance, in a neutral rather than emotional manner. Using this detached observation as a platform/springboard, the meditator can succeed in harnessing/tethering the distracted and agitated mind and bring it to a state of steadiness and tranquility so that calm reappraisal of the mind can be possible. This is called the *mindfulness-based detached monitoring* (MBDM; Pradhan et al., 2019) which makes it possible for the liberating cognitions (Pali. *nana*) and meditative insight and wisdom (Pali. *vipassana*) to ensue. An analogy may elucidate further the state of detachment. Let's imagine a scenario in which an old car stopped in the middle of a traffic and the driver desperately

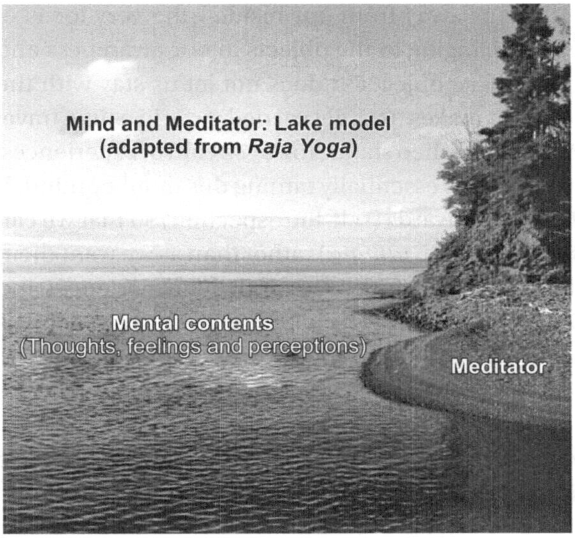

- All experiences are just elaborations of the **FIVE COMPONENTS by the mind**
- **Mind and meditators** are **different** from each other
- Meditation is **DETACHED OBSERVATION** of the mind (the five components): This gives rise to **Insight**
- Meditation needs **Philosophy + Techniques** + Practice (TRILOGY)
- MIDDLE WAY (Path of moderation) is the meditative life style

Fig. 3: Mind versus Meditator: *Detached observation* of the five-factors is meditation.

tries to get it moving. If he does so by pushing it from inside, it will not move. He definitely needs to step outside of the car and push it from there. This 'stepping outside' is the state of detachment: it is 'watching mind from a distance', a reflective process, so that one gets insight into the workings of the complex mind. **Figure 3** provides an illustrated summary of meditation.

Attaining a detached state of mind is a prerequisite for the meditator to ascend further in the meditation journey and to attain the higher level of meditative states. These states are essentially different grades of altered consciousness. Without achieving these meditative states, meditation practice is just a ritual or driven-doing (striving) rather than a direct experience or a state of being. Once the detached states of the mind are attained, the practitioner's attention becomes *wide open, yet detached* from the objects of the world: the mind become quite alert yet relaxed; open, inclusive and supple; receptive and responsive rather than reactive. In this mindfulness-based detached monitoring (MBDM) of all the objects in one's awareness (both internal and external), the observation becomes an effortless awareness where everything is perceived as peaceful, *as they are* (Pali. *tathata*). In such a state, there is complete acceptance, complete harmony—no need to change anything.

I will sum up this section by stating that, the timeless wisdom of the Yogic philosophies informs us on the *fundamental things* about the *modus operandi* of the human mind which form the basis for their psychotherapeutic use. The basic property of the mind is *distraction* and *projection*. It is a *monkey mind*

(Wei-an, 2000): it constantly runs away from our inside—the very locus of all our experiences. It keeps on clinging to the objects in our awareness and makes us (mis-) identify with these objects. It does not let us stay with the true experience of the moment, it makes us to get carried away in a time travel mode rather than maintaining a detached stance to our stream of experiences. Meditation—a central step of Yoga, is essentially taming this monkey mind. It is the process of turning the mind inwards (self-introspection) so that we can realize our experiences *as they are* (Pali. *tathata*) rather than as we want them to be. Because our inside (i.e., the mind) is the seat of all our experiences and mental phenomena (Sanskrit. *chitta-vritti*), it is paramount to study one's inside, to gain insight (inner knowledge) so that these experiences can be calmly noticed (detached observation) and clearly comprehended. From this clear comprehension (Pali. *sampajjana*), the *right view* (Sanskrit. *samyak dristi*) emerges and *wisdom* ensues. This is possible by deep contemplative practices such as meditation. These are the deep rationale for the therapeutic and stress-ameliorating effects of Yoga and meditation.

YOGA AND MINDFULNESS-BASED COGNITIVE THERAPY (Y-MBCT): A SUMMARY

The rationale for use of Yoga and meditation for self-analysis and psychotherapy is based on two major pragmatic concepts elaborated in the scriptural traditions of ancient India and mentioned below:

1. Yoga as a profound psychosomatic science that informs us about the deep influences of the mind on our body, and how to prepare the body and mind for meditation by using the steps 1 to 5 of the *Eight-limbed Yoga*.
2. Meditation as a science to cultivate stable states of attention (Concentration; Pali. *samatha*). Central importance of attention and awareness in meditation can be appreciated when one examines the original Pali term for mindfulness, i.e., *satipatthana* (*sati* means 'attention and awareness', *upatthana* means 'placing nearby' or 'making it ready at hand'). So, the literal meaning of mindfulness is "attending with awareness" (Analayo, 2003. p. 29). For the meditator, concentration acts as a raft to watch the mental contents (five factors of the mind) and mental phenomena with full awareness, in a clam and detached manner. This is mindfulness (Pali. *Vipassana* method) and the goal is to gain insight—to access the inner knowledge about self so that wisdom blossoms.

Taking these philosophies into account, the Yoga and mindfulness-based cognitive therapy (Y-MBCT) models emphasize the use of Yoga not in piecemeal, but *in its entirety*, i.e., all eight limbs that include meditation and meditative life style (Buddha's *Middle Way;* Pali. *Majhima magga;* Sanskrit.

Madhyamaka; Dalai Lama 2009). The eight-stepped methods are already described in the previous section and here I will provide a brief description of the *Middle Way*. To be meditative, one needs some basic preparations that includes the cultivation of a meditative lifestyle and a balanced view of life: that is essentially the *Middle Way*. It provides the necessary environment or nurturing matrix in which the meditative states blossom and flourish. It creates in us an ongoing and nonjudgmental awareness of self and life. This simple awareness redirects us toward the middle, that's why the name is the Middle Way: the path of moderation. Buddha's *Middle Way* is the path of *moderation* and *compassion*. This is the path that helps to pull ourselves from the extreme states and *center us* for our wellbeing. To live the Middle Way is analogous to driving in the middle lane in a road with three lanes —the other two lanes are in the extremes and do not give us any room if a change or adaptation is needed. Being the path of moderation and compassion, the Middle Way style keeps our meditation practice centered rather than creating extreme states such as self-criticality or striving to do the 'perfect meditation'. This awareness appraises us of the extreme nature inherent in our thoughts, feelings, perceptions, and actions of our daily lives—the sources of stress and sufferings. As realized and exemplified by the Buddha in his own life, the Middle Way gives us the inner tranquility and meditative bliss in the midst of the endless actions of daily life. From this, blossoms the insight (Pali. *nana*, Sanskrit. *jnana*). This insight and wisdom, when added to the actions of daily life, paves the way for self-awakening and liberation from the sufferings co-created by the five-factors of the mind (Dalai Lama, 2009). The constellation of the Middle Way choices to dwell our life meaningfully may be all that stands between us and a meditative life of acceptance, totality, bliss and self-actualization. Without incorporation of the Middle Way philosophy, meditation practice runs the risk of becoming just a set of empty rituals, without getting *realized* or incorporated into our daily lives in meaningful ways.

The Y-MBCT models are adapted from and inspired by the philosophies and praxes of the three original scriptural schools of Yoga and mindfulness, i.e., the Eight-Limbed Yoga (*Ashtanga*) of Patanjali (circa. 400 BC), the mindfulness (*satipatthana*) method of the Buddha (circa. 6th century BC), and the standardizations burrowed from the technique-rich style of *Tantra*, the most modern school of Yoga (circa. 2nd century CE) (detailed in a monograph: Pradhan, 2014). Their fidelity to the original scriptural traditions of Yoga and their amalgamation with the evidence-based pragmatic formats of the Western psychotherapy (cognitive behavioral- and psychodynamic/object relational psychotherapies), make them truly 'fusion models' of treatment. Since their inception in 1998, Pradhan and colleagues have tested the clinical efficacies of the Y-MBCT models in many research trials in disorder specific ways—as monotherapies as well as in combination with medications and neuromodulation interventions (Pradhan, 2014; Pradhan et al., 1998, 2016–2020). Below is a brief mention of these models and their clinical indications. Detailed descriptions of them are beyond the scope of this chapter and can be found in our other work (published and unpublished). The Y-MBCT models are disorder specific *(illness models)* and are extension of the *Standardized Meditation Program (StaMP), the wellness model.* Because establishing the meditation skills are a prerequisite before the patient is able to apply meditation for amelioration of the disorder specific psychopathologies or symptoms, *StaMP first ensures the meditation skill building in the patients* (and caregivers as well) by formal training in Yoga and meditation.

As disorder specific models, the Y-MBCT (*illness models*) cover most of the DSM-5 disorders as outlined below (detailed in Pradhan, 2014; Pradhan et al., 1998, 2016–2020):

- *TIMBER* (*Trauma Interventions* using *Mindfulness Based Extinction* and *Reconsolidation* of memories) serves as a prototype of the Y-MBCT fusion models which has been efficacious in treatment of chronic post-traumatic stress disorder (PTSD), treatment resistant depression, traumatic psychosis, borderline personality disorder, panic disorder, and generalized anxiety disorder (Pradhan et al., 2019). TIMBER has two specialized modifications for two difficult to treat conditions:
    - *TIMBER-AM (TIMBER Addiction Module):* For treatment of *addiction* (Chemical and Behavioral)
    - *TIMBER-PM (TIMBER Pain Module):* For treatment of *chronic pain*
- *Mindfulness-Based Graded Exposure and Response Modification (MB-GERM):* For treatment of obsessive-compulsive disorder (OCD)
- *Mindfulness-Based Rehabilitation of Reading, Attention and Memory (MBR-RAM):* For treatment of *cognitive disorders, dyslexia, ADHD*
- *Mindfulness-Based Cognitive Therapy, Insomnia module* ($MBCT_i$): For treatment of insomnia
- *Mindfulness-Based Cognitive Therapy, Eating disorder module* ($MBCT_e$): For treatment of eating disorders.

In the Y-MBCT models, the therapist practices Yoga and meditation with the patients during the therapy sessions. This prerequisite preserves the experiential essences of these models so that these do not end up becoming just jargon of words between the patient and therapist. Following the eight-stepped methods described before, these practices involve one's body (postures and bodily sensations), breathing, life style modifications, and training to achieve mastery on contemplation of *the five objects of the mind,* i.e., the thoughts, feelings, sensations/perceptions, will/desire/urges, and memories. The training of the patients on the four main aspects of the Y-MBCT models is mentioned below and is done in 10-sessions (30–45 minutes each):

1. *Achieving the concentration states:* This involves training on practice of sustained attention (*concentration* or Buddha's *sensate meditation* methods). This is done by use of Yogic postures (Sanskrit. *asana*) and Yogic praxes (Sanskrit. *kriya*) that includes *trataka,* a concentration method using the visual cues. This training is done over *two sessions* using initially the breath as the meditation object (attentional anchor, Pali. *kasina*) followed by generalization to the nonbreath objects or any physical sensations as the attentional anchor to stabilize the attention (Pradhan, 2014; Pradhan et al., 2020).
2. *Practice of the Middle Way:* Training on the Middle Way is done over *one session* by applying the *STOPP* module to the stressful daily life situations. STOPP module is the behavioral equivalent of the Middle Way, a paradigm developed by Pradhan (Pradhan et al., 2019. Pp. 73–75). It is the acronym for *S* = stop, *T* = three/ten/twenty breaths depending on the need, *O* = observe, *P* = planning for next steps/practice more, *P* = proceed ahead. Once trained, patients are encouraged to apply it during their *routine practice* (for meditation skill building) and *as needed practice* (for applying meditation skills to the daily life situations as they come).
3. *Attainment of the mindful states:* Training on this is done over *two sessions* by using the *meditation road map* and the *staged meditation protocols* (SMPs) standardized by Pradhan (2014).
4. *Mindfulness-based CBT:* Once meditation skills are established by the previous three steps, patient is trained over 4–6 sessions about how to apply the mindful states for cognitive reappraisal and reformulation of the symptoms and dysfunctions using disorder-specific cognitive behavioral therapy (CBT) modules. Apart from the cognitive reappraisal method, the mindfulness-based graded exposure therapy (MB-GET, Pradhan et al., 2019. p. 37–38) is a main CBT technique used in all Y-MBCT modules. The MB-GET method empowers the individual and reduces the dysfunctions by decreasing the anxiety, avoidance and arousal responses in the various trigger situations of daily life.

Using the real-time EEG biofeedback methods, Pradhan has standardized the meditation practice into *skill-levels 1 to 5* and *practice levels 1 to 10,* in order of increasing sophistications (Pradhan et al., 2019. pp. 39–40). Once the patient has attained the meditation *skill-level 3 and practice level 5* (which usually happens in 4–5 sessions), he/she is encouraged to apply the Y-MBCT models in disorder-specific ways to target the psychopathologies and the associated dysfunctions. Because the therapist practices Yoga and meditation with the patients during the therapy sessions, these aspects get facilitated.

TIMBER AS A PROTOTYPE OF THE Y-MBCT FUSION MODELS

TIMBER (*T*rauma *I*nterventions using *M*indfulness *B*ased *E*xtinction and *R*econsolidation of memories) psychotherapy is a novel, evidence-based, and biomarker-informed mindfulness-based CBT approach developed by Pradhan to address some of the existing treatment gaps in many chronic psychiatric conditions such as chronic post-traumatic stress disorder (PTSD), treatment-resistant depression, traumatic psychosis, chronic addiction and borderline personality disorder (Pradhan et al., 2019). TIMBER is a *translational, targeted,* and *time limited* therapy *(the three Ts of TIMBER)* that combines the experiential aspects of the Yoga and mindfulness with the pragmatism and targeted approaches of CBT. Technically, TIMBER belongs to the emerging category of the *third wave of CBT* (Kahl et al., 2012). Initially developed for treatment of chronic PTSD and subsequently applied to other disorders, TIMBER serves as a prototype of the Y-MBCT fusion models and has been tested efficacious in many randomized controlled trials (Pradhan et al., 2017, 2018). The plasma concentration of D-serine (an amino acid) has been used as a biomarker of response to TIMBER therapy (Pradhan et al., 2018). TIMBER involves a broad array of many psychotherapeutic components. In addition to incorporating the mindfulness-based tools, TIMBER involves the use of modified CBT interventions, such as mindfulness-based graded exposure therapy (MB-GET) and *cognitive reformulation and reprocessing* of the distressing memories in less emotional ways by use of the mindful states that have been attained by the use of standardized Yoga-meditation protocols. Although the evidence base for CBT is quite strong for a broad range of psychiatric conditions, CBT has important caveats as well, mostly in terms of patient engagement in the therapeutic process. Due to the format inherent to it, CBT often overemphasizes on the need for achieving the treatment goals in a time limited manner which can create unhealthy states especially when patients are not ready, such as feelings of ineptness and striving, thus creating additional stress and contributing to patient drop outs. In the traditional cognitive-behavioral trauma therapy, the use of relational principles and techniques are not yet common, and the therapist attunement and empathy are not always highly valued. These can pose as barriers to patient engagement. Similarly, although psychodynamic approaches do have a relational focus, more often than not, they are not time limited and therapy titration (dosing) are usually considered as not that important. One of the criticisms leveled against psychotherapy today, particularly CBT, is for the process being too technical with less emphasis on the experience which in turn may reduce the patient engagement into the therapeutic process, more so in trauma therapy. Taking these issues into considerations, the psychotherapeutic processes in TIMBER try to strike a balance with respect to these important limitations in the existing trauma therapy. In its evidence-based format, TIMBER uses two mechanisms of learning and memories to change the expression of traumatic memories, i.e., *extinction* of the traumatic memories and *reconsolidation* of calming memories: hence the name is TIMBER. In TIMBER, the use of these two memory mechanisms in a balanced combination contributes to the reduction of over-flooding in patients, enhances their skill-building process as well as engagement in the therapeutic process and this explains its therapeutic robustness. Of note, many contemporary trauma therapies (e.g., prolonged exposure therapy) use extinction-only approach which has important patient engagement limitations in addition to mechanistic caveats. Extinction, unlike reconsolidation, just suppresses the memories rather than updating them. Also, extinction is a context-dependent process, i.e., if the boundary conditions of exposure change, the therapy may fail. These important limitations of the extinction-only approaches can lead to quicker relapse in new settings of trauma and related triggers.

TIMBER uses a two-staged approach: the initial *wellness model* for meditation skill-building and the subsequent *illness-/disorder-specific* model for addressing the core psychopathologies and the associated dysfunctions. The skill building in the client and caregivers is done by their formal training in Yoga and meditation by the *Standardized Meditation Program* (*StaMP,* Pradhan et al., 2019) which forms its *wellness component.* This training takes 2–4 sessions, done at a frequency of once a week, 30–45 minutes duration each. Once the patients have attained the meditation *skill-level 3* and *practice level 5* (which usually happens in 4–5 sessions), they are encouraged to specifically focus on systematically changing the expressions of traumatic memories in their daily life situations by use of the two main CBT methods described above (i.e., mindfulness-based graded exposure therapy and cognitive reappraisal/cognitive reformulations using the already cultivated mindful states). TIMBER has two versions: Full TIMBER and mini-TIMBER (i.e., the STOPP module, described before). The full TIMBER is the longer version of TIMBER and consists of 15–20 minutes of the therapy session that entails exposure using the MB-GET methods followed by reappraisal: this promotes extinction of the traumatic memories. The mini-TIMBER is the shorter version that consists of 5–10 minutes of meditation using the STOPP module and promotes reconsolidation of the calming memories and cognitive reformulations. Mini-TIMBER specifically helps the patients to quickly de-escalate the arousal symptoms as they arise spontaneously in their daily life situations in response to trauma-related cues/triggers. TIMBER uses controlled reactivation of trauma memories for effective reconsolidation of the memories (updating the trauma memories) rather than over-flooding by using a specific scale, the *Arousal Response to Trauma Memory Reactivation* (ART-MR, Pradhan et al., 2019, Chap. 4). Thus, by the ongoing use of both

Full TIMBER and mini-TIMBER, subsequent calm and detached reappraisal of expressions of trauma memories is achieved, and new learning becomes possible in the patients to assist them in their recovery.

CONCLUSION

Drawing extensively from the neurobiology, traditional and applied psychology and spiritual psychology, the Y-MBCT fusion models are Pradhan's humble attempts to bridge some of the existing treatment gaps in many neuropsychiatric conditions. The Y-MBCT methods have been used as standalone therapies as well as in combination with other psychotherapies or medications or brain stimulation methods for treatment of the various neuropsychiatric conditions. As far as testing the clinical efficacy of disorder specific and targeted treatment approaches are concerned, these are relatively unexplored areas in psychology and psychiatry and lot more needs to be done to ameliorate these important health conditions. Our clinical and research work are ongoing in these aspects and we hope to keep our readers informed in future.

FURTHER READING

1. Analayo. Satipatthana: The direct path to realization. Windhorse Publications, Birmingham, UK; 2003.
2. Aurobindo. The synthesis of Yoga. The complete works of Sri Aurobindo. Sri Aurobindo Ashram Publication Department: Pondicherry, India. 1999;23-24.
3. Beck AT. Cognitive therapy and the emotional disorders. New York: International University Press; 1976.
4. Bion WR. Notes on memory and desire. Psychoanal Forum. 1967;2(3):271-80.
5. Bodhi B. The Noble Eightfold Path: Way to the end of suffering. Onalaska, WA: Pariyatti Publications; 2000.
6. Dalai Lama. The Middle Way: Faith Grounded in Reason. Wisdom Publications, Sommerville, MA, USA; 2009.
7. Eliade M. Yoga: For Immortality and Freedom, 2nd edition. Princeton University Press: Princeton, New Jersey; 1969.
8. Feuerstein G. Encyclopedic dictionary of Yoga. Paragon House Print: New York, NY; 1990.
9. Feuerstein, G. The Yoga Tradition: Its History, Literature, Philosophy and Practice, 3rd edition. Hohm Press: Prescott, AZ; 2001.
10. Feuerstein, G. The Yoga-Sutra of Patanjali. A New Translation and Commentary. Inner Traditions International. Rochester, VT; 1979.
11. Frawley D. Yoga and Ayurveda: Self-healing and Self-realization. Lotus Press: Wisconsin; 1999.
12. Freud S. In: The Unconscious (J. Strachey, Trans.). Standard edition of the complete psychological works of Sigmund Freud. The Hogarth Press: London, UK. 1915;14.

13. Gunaratana B. Beyond Mindfulness in Plain English. Wisdom Publications; Sommerville, MA: USA; 2009.
14. Ingram, DM. Mastering the core teachings of the Buddha: An unusually hardcore. Dharma book. Aeon Books Ltd., London NW3: UK; 2008.
15. Kahl KG, Winter L, Schweiger U. The third wave of cognitive behavioral therapies. Current Opinions in Psychiatry. 2012;25(6):522-8.
16. Lazarus RS, Alfert E. Short-circuiting of threat by experimentally altering cognitive appraisal. Journal of Abnormal Psychology. 1964;69:195-205.
17. Lutz A, Brefczynski-Lewis J, Johnstone T, Davidson R. Regulation of the neural circuitry of emotion by compassion meditation: effects of meditative expertise. PLoS One. 2008;3(3):1897.
18. Nanamoli B. The Middle Length Discourses (Majjhima Nikaya) of the Buddha: BPS Publications, Kandy, Sri Lanka; 1995.
19. Nanamoli B. The Path of Purification (Visuddhimagga): BPS Publications, Kandy, Sri Lanka; 1956.
20. Nyanaponika T. The Heart of Buddhist Meditation. Samuel Weiser, Inc., York Beach, ME: USA; 1954.
21. Pradhan B. Yoga and Mindfulness Based Cognitive Therapy: A Clinical Guide. Springer, Gewerbestrasse, Cham, Switzerland; 2014.
22. Pradhan BK, Malik S. Chapter-4: Yoga and mindfulness-based cognitive behavioral therapy for insomnia (Y-MBCTi). In: Sedky K, Nazir R, Bennett D (Eds). Sleep medicine and mental health: A guide for psychiatrists & other healthcare professionals. Springer International Publishing AG, Cham, Switzerland; 2020. ISBN:978-3-030-44446-4.
23. Pradhan BK, Mishra B (1998; unpublished data on 18-patients). A pilot project on utility of Yoga and meditation in a population with alcohol and opiate addiction. Research study conducted at the SCB, Medical College, India; 1998.
24. Pradhan BK, Mitrev L, Moaddel R, Wainer I. D-Serine is a biomarker for clinical response in (R, S)-ketamine treatment of post-traumatic stress disorder and co-morbid depression. Biochim Biophys Acta (BBA-Proteins and Proteomics). 2018;1866(7):831-9.
25. Pradhan BK, Parikh T, Sahoo M, Selznick R, Goodman M. Current understanding of dyslexia and pilot data on efficacy of MBR-RAM (Mindfulness Based Rehabilitation of Reading, Attention & Memory) therapy model. Adolescent Psychiatry; 2017. pp. 44-55.
26. Pradhan BK, Pinninti NR. Chapter-5. Yoga & mindfulness based cognitive therapy for psychosis (Y-MBCTp): A pilot study on its efficacy as brief therapy. In: Pradhan, Pinninti and Rathod (Eds). Brief Interventions for psychosis: A Clinical Compendium. Springer Publishers, Switzerland; 2016.
27. Pradhan BK, Pinninti NRP, Rathod SR. TIMBER Psychotherapy: For PTSD, Depression and Traumatic Psychosis. Springer, Gewerbestrasse, Cham, Switzerland; 2019.
28. Pradhan BK. Chapter-13. Psychiatric Aspects in Chronic Pain and Utility of Yoga and Mindfulness Based Cognitive Behavioral Therapy for Pain (Y-MBCT-pain) as a Translational Model. In: Sabia M, Sehdev J, Bentley W (Eds). Urogenital Pain: A Clinicians Guide to Diagnosis and Interventional Treatments. Springer Publishers, Switzerland; 2017. ISBN: 978-3-319-30519-6.

29. Reddy MS. Psychotherapy—insights from Bhagavad Gita. Indian J Psychol Med. 2012;34:100-4.
30. Santina PD. The Tree of Enlightenment: An introduction to the major traditions of Buddhism. Buddha Dharma Education Association Inc., Chico, CA: USA; 1997.
31. Satchidananda S. The Yoga Sutras of Patanjali: translations and commentary. Integral Yoga Publications, Yogaville, VA, USA; 1978.
32. Seligman MEP, Csikszentmihalyi M. 'Positive Psychology: An Introduction". American Psychologist. 2000;55 (1):5-14.
33. Taimni IK. The science of Yoga: the Yoga-sutras of Patanjali. Nesma Books, India; 1961.
34. Tang Y-Y, Holzel BK, Posner MI. The neuroscience of mindfulness meditation. Nat Rev Neurosci. 2015;16:213-25.
35. Venkoba Rao A. Bhagavad Gita and psychotherapy. Bhavan's Journal; 1978. pp. 19-23, 35-38.
36. Wei-an C. Taming the monkey mind: A guide to pure land practice. Buddha Dharma Education Association Inc., New York: NY; 2000.
37. Yogananda P. God talks with Arjuna: The Bhagavad Gita: Royal Science of God Realization. Yogoda Satsanga Society, Dakshineswar, Calcutta: India; 1995.

9

CHAPTER

An Immigrant Indian Psychiatrist's Journey to become a Medical Psychotherapist

Nitesh Painuly

ABSTRACT

In the predominantly 'medicalized' model of British psychiatry, it is quite unusual for a General Psychiatrist to forge a career in psychotherapy. The choice is even more striking for a young immigrant physician from India. The initially floundering, then blossoming, and finally consolidating and rewarding steps of such a journey are described in this chapter. The turmoil borne by its author involved not only considerable new learning but also a gradual and important shift in his core identity. This was facilitated by his finding a significant mentor and by his participation in group therapeutic work.

Keywords: Medical Psychotherapist, Culture, Identity

INTRODUCTION

Traditionally in United Kingdom (UK), a psychiatrist specializing in psychotherapy has been called a 'Consultant Psychotherapist', akin to 'Consultant Psychiatrist' and at the same time ambiguous enough to keep its nonmedical stance alive. Still, in the National Health Service (NHS) in UK, within the hierarchy of psychotherapy, and psychiatry both, consultant psychotherapist held a somewhat admired (at times envied), mythical and mystical position. I remember attending a day workshop run by a prominent Kleinian analyst; who, in reminiscing about his old days, mentioned that as a consultant psychotherapist, one took a couple of schizophrenic patients for 5 days a week analysis and that was an whole career's worth of clinical work. Today, the theoretical stance is relatively noncommittal; though traditionally it had psychoanalytic/psychodynamic stances and there are growing numbers of consultant psychotherapists, who represent group therapy, cognitive behavioral therapy (CBT), and systemic family therapy. Though my impression about this large group is that an implicit hierarchy exits in it whereby psychoanalysts are at the top, psychoanalytic informed therapists in the middle, and the rest are not in either of these two leagues.

The role of consultant psychotherapist has also changed. In an increasingly regulated and limited budget NHS, most of the psychotherapy work is provided through nonmedical professionals, i.e., clinicians from nursing, social work, psychology and educational background who do further training in psychotherapy. Most of the therapists and counselors are of CBT and other nonanalytic therapy orientation probably due to shorter training and greater demand for this kind of work.

An important development in NHS psychotherapy counseling scene is the 2008 implementation of the Integrated Access to Psychological Treatment (IAPT) program across England. IAPT is a national-level dissemination program for provision of evidence-based psychological treatments (mainly CBT) for anxiety and depression in the UK. IAPT was founded in the context of global financial crises and on the premise that many patients receiving an evidence-based psychological therapy would likely recover and return to work, therefore reducing the welfare benefit cost burden (Clark, 2011). It is a good example of how even in difficult times new and innovative ideas can come to fruition if they fit-in with the existing socio-political agenda. Today, IAPT with around more than 200 centers across England and with 1.25 million annual referrals is the largest publicly funded and systematic implementation of evidence-based psychological care in the world. Recent meta-analysis (Wakefield et al., 2021) shows IAPT interventions are associated with large treatment effect sizes in depression and anxiety and moderate effect with regards to work and social adjustment. This can be considered one of the legacy of NHS, where everyone can easily get a limited number of counseling sessions for minor mental disorders.

At the same time, a 2005 guidance issued by the Department of Health under the title of 'New Ways of Working for Psychiatrists' noted the increasing difficulty in filling posts of consultant psychotherapists. The same report showed that among all subspecialties psychotherapy had the lowest number of consultants and the lowest increase in the employment rate in last 5 years. Even the trainees who had done psychotherapy training were returning to do other forms of specialty training for better prospects of employment; psychotherapy was labeled a 'dying specialty'.

In this changed context, it is not surprising that the endangered breed of consultant psychotherapist was re-branded as 'Medical Psychotherapist' by the Department of Health endorsement of the Royal College of Psychiatrists. The specialty of 'Psychotherapy' was re-named as 'Medical Psychotherapy' (Mace and Healy, 2011) in order to differentiate psychiatrists with psychotherapy training and their responsibilities from nonmedical psychotherapists. It was also intended to enhance public credibility since medical psychotherapists would be regulated by the General Medical Council (the governing body for all physicians in the UK), whereas nonmedical therapists would have a rather elusive and unclear accreditation process. However, to have 'officially' delineated a role is hardly equal to defining an internal sense of identity. As the Kakars (2009) put it:

> "Identity is not a role, with which it is often confused. It is not a garment that can be put on or taken off according to the weather outside; it is not 'fluid,' but marked by a sense of continuity and sameness irrespective of where the person finds himself during the course of his life" (p. 1).

I do not think there is a description of his or her identity which will suit every 'Medical Psychotherapist', as each has his or her own unique journey which forms their identity through the unique course of their life. For me, it goes to the question, who essentially I am at work?: A doctor, ? a psychiatrist, ? a psychotherapist? When I use title of 'Consultant Psychiatrist in Medical Psychotherapy' do I mean a specific kind of psychiatrist? Or a specific kind of therapist? Or both? Or neither?

MY JOURNEY

I grew-up in a town called Uttarkashi in the northern state of Uttarakhand in India. Being raised by driven parents and choosing medicine as a career was hardly a surprise. However, my complete unpreparedness for becoming a doctor is captured by the fact that upon entering the King Georges' Medical College in Lucknow in 1993, I was surprised to find out that I had to learn human anatomy and physiology for this course. I was scared and unsure during my medical school years and tried to do what seemed to be the 'right' thing, essentially was to get into a one of the popular subspecialties of that time. I was lucky that we had a good placement in psychiatry. It was required that we attend that placement regularly (an early lesson on how structure is important before any effective learning can happen!). I remember one particular lecture on Freud made a particular impression on me, where probably first time I realized that medicine could be fun. Overall during my undergraduate years I learned the ropes and I worked hard enough to ultimately secure a rank in the Postgraduate Institute of Medical Education and Research ('PGI' in short) in Chandigarh, which did not offer me the specialty I wanted; psychiatry was the only realistic option left.

In my years as a psychiatry resident, I somehow survived the academic rigor of the department. It took me about a year to drop my stethoscope (literally and metaphorically) and accept that my tools were really listening, and learning when and how to speak. Compared to other institutes in psychiatry in India, in PGI there was an acknowledgment of psychoanalytic thinking and an attempt to continue to learn it through case formulation, and with some clinical work under supervision. Some of the psychotherapy work which I still remember from those days was my treating a patient with 'hysteria' (which was my first exposure to the gratifying experience of positive transference) and also an unsuccessful and frustrating work with a borderline patient.

When time came to choose the topic of my dissertation, I was lucky to have a research guide who gave me many ideas as well as freedom to choose my topic. I decided to test the psychoanalytic hypothesis of depression as 'anger turned inwards'. My fascination with 'anger' would make further sense later when I migrated from India and found myself full of rage and hurt (which had been well-defended and managed so far). This probably was the main driving force for me to go for psychoanalytic training which meant arranging a therapy for myself (perhaps the only way I could accept treatment for myself at that time).

For first 5 years in England, I just survived. In an act of 'unmentalized' wisdom, I joined group supervision offered by the psychotherapy department during my first year of immigration. I was struggling to make sense of my new status as an 'immigrant' in a strange country; there was also the struggle with a sense of guilt and shame at having left my 1-year-old daughter behind in India. And when she joined us, I was not sure how to relate with her and felt completely lost. It was in such circumstances that I started my training in psychodynamic psychotherapy arranging my personal therapy, supervision and psychotherapy cases. In a paper that I was soon required to write (Painuly, 2008), I described my personal encounter with 'causality' in psychoanalytic thinking.

> "I have struggled a great deal with the issue of causality (in my therapy). Whenever my therapist would make a link between my current problems and my past, I would try to resist it (I still do). It would be painful to see that my current suffering has just been reduced to the past. I would argue, what is immediate or obvious, is not being addressed which I thought was the real cause. I would find my therapist's emphasis excessive and an overreaction and I would put this difficulty down to my therapist's lack of understanding of our cultural differences. I was fighting with my therapist over the issue of causality and gradually I started losing this battle. First, I noticed myself seeing some themes and associations around and I was becoming more tolerant of the therapist interpretations. Secondly, I was getting less tormented by this issue of what is causing what. Despite continuing to resist these connections intellectually, just the awareness of them was causing 'something' in a very experiential domain (which itself was new experience for me). It was like wires were getting connected and the 'current' deep down which was obstructed so far, had started flowing. Not that my therapist was right about my problems, but it was very much the experience of finding the meaning or getting that glimpse of a possibility of finding meaning, which was reducing my fixation on coming up with some definitive cause" (p.11).

For first 3 years in therapy, all I did was to offer myself to the therapist as a patient who was a consultant psychiatrist, intellectually capable, and 'a good patient'. Despite all the attempts to control my therapist and my therapy, it was proving quite difficult; and breaks in therapy were especially painful and somewhat bewildering when I would see myself acting out in ways which would surprise me. During this difficult period what kept me going was a good and stimulating academic program and my almost addictive love of psychoanalytic literature. More than the understanding of what I was reading, it was the experience of reading itself that gratified me; I was like a baby in a crib and was being fed. This was a unique and almost pleasantly dissociative experience. Bion and Fairbairn especially became my heroes, not only because of their writing but also owing to the kind of life they had led. Bion was born in India and this colonial connection had some special meaning for me. Fairbairn, though Scottish, would come into my dreams as an Indian, helping me walk along a bridge that other people seem to be crossing with ease. I tried to make sense of this in one of my term papers on 'Regression' (Painuly, 2009).

> "When I began my personal therapy, there was a fear in me that I could have a psychotic breakdown through therapy. Gradually therapy started progressing and I could see some behavior emerging in myself, which I hadn't expected. I started finding myself very vulnerable. Until this term, I was not taking it either as a regression or progression. It was simply like looking at the other side of me which I was not aware of so far. I was frustrated by this, but at the same time assured that my therapist does not find it unexplainable and someway she was expecting it to emerge" (p. 9).

This paper, alongside my reading of Little's (1985)[1] essay on regression, transformed my initial fear of psychotic breakdown into a romantic longing for it. As I started reading more on regression, a desire in me started growing up to go through some big 'regressive' spell. I was getting more and more preoccupied with having a 'basic fault' (Balint, 1968) within me which needed to be completely exposed before getting restructured. I started thinking of this as a quick fix solution of my problems, in the same way as some patients wished for brain surgery as the ultimate cure of their longstanding emotional difficulties. I started attending each session with a hope that this time something is going to happen; may be I would do a somersault leading to a 'new beginning'.[2] Gradually, I came to realize my narcissistic needs, where even my 'basic fault' has to be big'. I had to live with my own mild, nagging (but painful) regression and I had to own it. At the same time, I started

[1]This paper is about the analysand's prospective on Winnicott's approach of dealing with the psychotic regression. In my view, this is a very powerful and moving personal account but difficult to generalize to the routine practice of psychoanalysis.

[2]On regression, Balint (1968) describes a case, where a young lady, who could never do somersaults spontaneously stands from the couch and takes a perfect somersault on the floor. Later, this proved to be a major breakthrough in her treatment.

realizing that I had been doing a few little somersaults of mental growth even without noticing them.

Exploring the psychotic aspect of my anxiety came lot later, when I had started working in an Early Intervention Service for Psychosis. Soon after finishing my personal therapy, I attended a 10 days silent Vipassana retreat. Though it was an intense experience and almost like a mini-crisis but this freed me from the fear of going mad. I found myself relating with my psychotic patients from a curious inquisitive place where I could go with them and could see the creativity inherent in madness. There was also a sense of sadness to see the cost of avoiding 'reality'. Managing two different roles of a psychiatrist and psychotherapist was a struggle most of the time. It was linked with my internal struggle to work out my real identity through these roles. This is reflected in my following case-history (Painuly, 2009).

Clinical Vignette 1

> Change of my role from her psychiatrist to psychotherapist was a loss for my patient, Mrs K and for myself as well. She started missing my reassuring and guiding role. Now, I was expecting her to take lead in the sessions, mostly silent and not giving 'straight' answers and this left Mrs K perplexed and frustrated. Her depression worsened and she wanted me to change her antidepressant, while I would try to direct her to more relevant issues with my all uncertainties and anxiety of a 'naïve' therapist. At this point, it became so difficult that Mrs K had to bring her husband for couple of her sessions and I ended up adding one more antidepressant, before we could proceed further. I also noticed that I would wear my ID batch when I am in session with Mrs K (usually, I take off my ID batch, when I see my psychotherapy patients). Clearly I was acting in out a counter-transference and giving reassurance to Mrs K (and to myself as well) that she hasn't lost her psychiatrist (p. 3).

Moving on to Group Work

I had some introduction to group work during my psychodynamic training. I had found it fascinating that there are invisible rules governing the group and its discourse, and that one could predict what might happen next if one observed the group carefully. But these were all ideas based on fantasy, until I come across Yvonne Agazarian's (1995) text; she is considered to Founder of Systems-Centered Training and Therapy. Only then I started learning seriously how to define and collect data, and develop and test hypotheses.

The dilemma of managing the conflict between being a therapist and a psychiatrist remained alive during my group therapy training. It became more marked when I felt that my employer, my team, and even my patients, wanted me to be a 'psychiatrist', and my being a 'therapist' was considered by them somehow my personal agenda. My group work would always be a topic of discussion in my job-planning meetings, which meant most of my therapy work I did was over and above my general adult consultant psychiatrist work, and in my personal time. I jotted some observation down at that time (Painuly, 2012).

> "I decided to start psychotherapy group in a team, where I had recently joined as a consultant psychiatrist. This team hadn't had a dedicated psychiatrist for last 5 years and overall was struggling from consistent clinical and managerial leadership. Though as a consultant I was welcomed in a team (and to great extent idealized) but at the same time when I mentioned about starting this group, response for support and patients referral was lukewarm. This also brought some suspiciousness esp. from other therapists within the teams. These two kind of different responses from the same team seemed confusing and only after sometime it occurred to me that the deal with team was to be a psychiatrist not a psychotherapist. This helped me to empathize with this kind of response and made me aware of the importance of keeping these two roles (e.g., psychiatrist vs. psychotherapist) separate in the context of my team" (p. 13).

In my group-analytic training, the main work I did was to make an isomorphic connection between individual and group and explore it through the structure and boundary of the group. In an essay I wrote during this time (Painuly, 2013), I explored the example of the suicide of one of my patients and attempted to link the individual and organizational dynamics.

Clinical Vignette 2

Ms J, a patient with borderline personality disorder was admitted to the acute psychiatric ward following an increased risk of suicide. She soon settled in the ward, started idealizing her psychiatrist, and expressing her views on a blog. Later she would express her devaluation and disappointments publicly through this blog. Ms J was never confronted directly with this boundary breach, but a sense of feeling exposed and vulnerable was quite evident among the staff. She would expect her assigned nurse to read her blog to find out how she was feeling, rather than discussing it in their one to one session.

Six weeks after admission, when Ms J was heading toward discharge, she killed herself by taking an overdose in the ward. The next couple of weeks were difficult in the ward, as expected. The police investigation into the incident made an overall sense of paranoia very real and tangible. Both the staff and patients were feeling angry but also trapped and helpless. The patients frequently acted out and sometimes they openly accused the staff for not being able to keep them safe and sometimes expressed their guilt at what they made the staff go through. The staff could only express their anger toward the management, and by not attending the staff support group meeting (when it was needed the most). The assigned nurse for this patient went off sick. In an internal enquiry into this incident, there were implicit suggestions that the treatment team should have been keeping an eye on the patient's blog as a way of policing her suicidal thoughts and managing the risk.

Acute in-patient units, considering the number of disturbed patients they house and the enormity of the tasks at their hands, are predisposed to turn into an antigroup (Nitsun, 1996) where all the destructiveness get projected into the group, without resources to assimilate them. Interestingly, it seems that management had an expectation of staff keeping a constant eye on a patient's blog (thoughts). This could be a reflection of a current culture of excessive emphasis on safety and risk management, but deep down this seems to be a narcissistic expectation of controlling everything, without any regard to individual boundaries as well as limitations. No wonder, both staff and patients were feeling trapped and helpless. Rosenfield (1987) in his conceptualization of 'gang' describes an internal process that seeks to obliterate need and dependency, by denying external reality and guards the inner self in a sadistic, controlling and omnipotent way, like the Mafia. This scenario confirms Nitsun (1996) when he maintains that "gang is a useful metaphor for the antigroup, suggesting a particular form of projective identification, in which an internalized destructive group is externalized and projected on to the real group" (p. 2).

In our group supervision, one of the supervisees, who runs a group in a prison setting, talked about the new entrant in her group. As the supervisee declared that this person has been in the newspaper quite a lot, because he murdered someone famous, the excitement and curiosity in the room was quite palpable. In a somewhat casual way, the identity of the murdered celebrity and also the prisoner was revealed. When I returned home, out of curiosity I started doing an internet search on this case and I soon found myself almost hooked on this whole incident. In a somewhat obsessive way, I started reading and looking for more information around this. My feelings at that time were a mix of excitement, fear, and also a sense of losing control. Only when I talked about this in personal therapy, did I recognize the boundary breach that had happened in our supervision? Suddenly it dawned on me; I was experiencing the same murderous rage toward my therapist, which was in context of ending of my therapy. This acknowledgment brought about a vigorous physical reaction (which I hadn't experienced before) and the closest name I could put on it was a mixture of rage and fear (p. 3).

THE NEXT DECADE

In next 8–9 years, I worked primarily with psychotic patients (as a consultant in early intervention in psychosis service) both as a psychiatrist and as a group therapist where we ran a weekly group called 'making sense'. I came to know the psychotic nature of group-work and how much it could get located in individuals (including the therapist). I also learned more about group-transferences.

Nonetheless, I felt a growing dissatisfaction with the group analytic approach. This brought me back with my battle with psychoanalytic thinking where the analyst (even group analyst) is the center of the universe, and genuine group-dynamic issues were in my view quite simplified by individual and group transference and if nothing worked than Foulksian quasi-mystical 'group-matrix' (Foulkes & Anthony, 1965) which could explain everything.

During the course of this training, I came across Yvonne Agazarian's (Agazarian & Gantt, 2000) work. A psychoanalyst in quest of finding a common language between group and individual work, Agazarian developed a theory of living human system; her systems-centered approach to the group work was based more on Lewinian approach (Lewin, 1951) of group dynamics than psychoanalytic.

I soon learned that Agazarian, who was in her eighties, came every year to England to run a week long intensive group experience training. I joined her first foundation group in 2014, thinking that I'd better meet her before she is unable to travel or passes away. This fear recurred every year when I would join her foundation group until 2018 when she passed away after 2 weeks of the last foundation group she did in York; I was lucky to be a part of that group and could say good-bye to her.

During the first group I attended with her, I knew I was back in the place where I needed to do more work on myself and, at the same time I felt somehow my analysis was complete. In my attempt to make sense of the weeks that followed, I emailed Agazarian and informed her of my inner conundrum. Her response was:

> "Dear Nitesh, in our Foundation Group, one of the teachings was called 'explaining vs. exploring': 'explaining' as a cognitive activity, which uses a different part of our brain from 'exploring'. Thus, we suggested that there are two sources of 'comprehension'. The first is 'words first and feelings second', and it is the thoughts that generate the feelings, not our 'exploratory researcher!' The second is 'exploration first and feelings second', and then we translate the information we get from our senses and emotions into words: this is our exploratory, researcher role. Korzybski said 'the map is not the territory'—implying that we have to keep checking our cognitive map against the real world and keep

revising it, which can be frustrating but helps us manage our life in the world of reality—and keeps our energy related to the universe" (personal communication, 15th November, 2015).

At this stage, I decided to change the course of my group training and I moved from group analysis to systems-centered training, which meant attending training group. Soon after that, I started my second spell of therapy, this time with a male therapist with systems-centered orientation. This time through my therapy and my training group, I learnt that my long-engrained character defenses in the context of my original family where they were perfect fit to keep the family system stable remain alive as they still serve many functions in my current family. I got very curious about my frequently taking 'scapegoat' role. Apart from family, this also does not make life easy of an immigrant in society which is rigid, stereotyped and racially prejudiced. And this time, I sent a long missive to the group.

"Dear Group, In SCT groups we don't scapegoat; instead, we find and join our subgroup of either scapegoat or scapegoater, and explore both sides of the conflict, one at a time. But what happens in non-SCT groups (which, by the way, happens to be the rest of the world)? Soon after working satisfactorily in an SCT group, I have found myself scapegoating another member in a 'nongroup' context, or, being scapegoated when I returned to my family context. Yes, I do see and observe myself doing a good scapegoat job and keep reminding myself of the universality of these human instincts. Still, I can't help behaving exactly as a scapegoat does; a 'lonely' act in a context, which is out of the context. I can almost hear Yvonne Agazarian saying to me something along these lines, "You see, you do this so you can say to the group 'Look, what you have done to me'" (a masochist drawing sadistic pleasure from his complaining). She probably would have said to the rest of the group, "Your version is, 'When we do this to you, it hurts us as well, but we do this for your own good'" (a sadist enjoying the masochistic pleasure).

Whilst I am attending my bruises from a recent deviant act, I have found the following two thoughts helpful. (1) Scapegoat (me) scapegoats the group, and the group (you) scapegoats the scapegoat, i.e., the scapegoat is a scapegoater at the same time. (2) There is not only one (me) deviant in the group; another one is called 'leader'. And you need both of us for your 'groupishness'. Your leader holds the system, I hold the structure. Your leader personifies communication, I personify noise. Your leader wants you to move toward your goal and I want you to deal with the problem (which is inevitable along the way). If you don't have either of us, you will either remain just a constellation of individuals or get jumbled up as a mass of 'herd'. My advice (in my wisdom of being

> a deviant) to you is to keep an eye on a deviant within you and keep asking him/her to join the 'leader' of that moment; who could be anyone including the leader you appointed, a self-proclaimed leader, a silent member or a raging deviant like me. And yes, despite being a deviant I continue to have a huge yearning for a good join!!" (Painuly, 2018).

Over the last 4 years of attending York Training weeks with Azagarian, I developed a small ritual with her. Every year, I will would buy one of her books from the training bookstall and will ask her to sign it for me. She would always oblige along with a personal message. These words with her own hand held a sense of sacredness for me like a '*Guru-mantra*' (In the Hindu spiritual tradition the Guru, or Master, gives his disciple a mantra in the form of a verbal, written, or nonverbal message/instruction, which the disciple keeps reflecting upon and pondering over again and again.). That's what these messages were for me: personal, with multiple layers of meaning, and something to work with for the whole year and beyond.

As this little exchange would take place usually on the 3rd day of the training week, there would invariably be the context of my own work in that week, and my relationship with Agazarian as a trainer.

In my second Foundation training group with Yvonne in 2015, I bought her magnum-opus *Systems-centered Therapy for Groups (1997)* during the lunch break and went straight into the afternoon session. It was a difficult session for me, and unbeknownst to me I was doing what I do in these circumstances. Yvonne was standing and writing something on the white board and I interrupted her again by asking a question. She turned around and gave me a fierce look and said, "Will you let me do the work with the group or will you keep interrupting me?" Further, she paused a while and added, "Do you realize how stubborn you are? And I have a hypothesis. This probably was the only way you could get any attention as a child." I was mortified and could not utter a single word for the rest of the session. However, once the session finished, I could muster the courage of asking her to sign my copy of *Systems-centered Therapy for Groups*. And Agazarian, without looking at me, wrote, "Nitesh, I'm afraid you will probably have to read this one over and over! I hope it's different each time! ☺ Yvonne."

That night was difficult. Though I could maintain enough curiosity to read the chapter from the book, *Resistance-to-Change Defenses*, where the stubbornness was discussed from an SCT point of view. Reading this made sense to me and it anchored me enough. It was like doing one to one work with Agazarian through her written words.

The next morning, before Agazarian joined the training, we as a group practiced "Undoing Role-Locks" protocol with the help of our co-leader. As a result, I felt freer and was able to resume my spontaneity. Once the session finished and as I was leaving for the break, I saw Yvonne walking into the room. Part of me was still angry with her (and also scared). I probably was intending to say a formal good morning and get out of her way as soon as I could. Nevertheless, Yvonne, with her inviting smile, stopped me and asked, "Have you unlocked your role this morning? Otherwise, I am going to spank you now!!" My spontaneous reply to her with a grinning smile was, "Yvonne, I am not going to give you any more trouble." At that moment, I felt a mixture of mischievousness and a sense of pride, just as a child would who has won a war between life and death with his mother. Also, her words were received as a medal for being a worthy opponent. Since then, I have read *Systems-centered Therapy for Groups* countless times, and as Agazarian had hoped, it always reveals different meanings each time (Painuly, 2020).

I am continuing to do training in systems-centered approach of group training that includes attending training group, doing skills training, theory work and one to one consultation. It is a different training though I check myself what I want to do, and what I am ready for rather than looking for any license at the end and sometime do more personal work in terms of therapy or more consultation work which include more supervision. When I have to prioritize my other areas of learning I take break from training group, and when I am ready to do further work, I join again. I have a sense of freedom and feel that I am moving gradually to building a bridge between individual and group work, east and west, and dualistic and nondualistic ways of looking at the 'reality.'

INTEGRATING SCIENCE AND PSYCHOLOGY

Systems-centered Training which is a theory-based tradition, re-kindled the dormant theoretician within me. This also brought forth genuine desire to practice 'science' as a discipline and use it as a tool.

Reading Kurt Lewin (1997) around this time came as a huge relief for me. He gave words to my underlying intuitive (but shaky) belief that social and psychological processes are as 'real' (and as 'unreal') as this physical material world is. Through his scientific rigor and research, he validated the reality of 'psychological field' (life space) as Einstein had with the existence of the 'gravitational field' (spacetime).

Lewin's concept of life-space and simplicity of its formulation is something I found extraordinarily beautiful. As Lewin (1997) says, the life space includes both the person and his psychological environment.

> "The task of explaining behavior then becomes identical with: (1) Finding a scientific representation of the life space (LSp) and (2) determining the function (F) which links the behavior to the life space. This function (F) is what one usually calls a law" (p. 338).

This is a very simple mathematical formula which Lewin (1997) explains in the following manner, in the context of groups:

> "Social events depend on the social field as a whole, rather than on a few selected items. This is the basic insight behind the field-theoretical method which has been successful in physics, which has steadily grown in psychology, and, in my opinion, is bound to be equally fundamental for the study of social fields, simply because it expresses certain basic characteristics of interdependence" (p. 338).

Further he writes:

> "Science tries to link certain observable (phenotypical) data with other observable data. It is crucial for all problems of interdependence, however, that-for reasons which we do not need to discuss here-it is, as a rule, impracticable to link one set of phenotypical data directly to other phenotypical data. Instead, it is necessary to insert "intervening variables". To use a more common language: The practitioner as well as the scientist views the observable data as mere 'symptoms'. They are 'surface' indications of some 'deeper lying' facts. He has learned to 'read' the symptoms, like a physicist reads his instruments. The equations which express physical laws refer to such deeper lying dynamic entities as pressure, energy, or temperature rather than to the directly observable symptoms such as the movements of the pointer of an instrument...While there is no need for social science to copy the specific concepts of the physical sciences, the social scientist should be clear that he, too, needs intervening variables and that these dynamic facts, rather than the external data and appearances, are the important points of reference alike for him and for the social practitioner". (p. 305)

In an attempt to relate Agazarian's theory of living human system and its practice, I wrote:

> "before the revised theory there was a lack of discrimination between Lewin's restraining force which is essentially the boundary condition (reality) and Yvonne's, restraining forces that are chasing the 'as if' goal (irreality). The closed boundary was mistakenly being confused with the restraining force. This is an important discrimination between what is driving/restraining and what is goal? And what is the relationship between them. For me, this is the moment when Agazarian's theory of Living Human Systems reveals its intervening variables, which Kurt Lewin had called worthy for every scientist to strive for" (Painuly 2021, p.15).

MAKING SENSE OF PSYCHOTHERAPY AS AN INDIAN IMMIGRANT

Comparing Western science as a discipline with Eastern spiritual traditions, in particular those of India, yields the following general points:

1. In contrary to scientific knowledge, where theories are empirical and falsifiable, in the spiritual way, there is an absolute reality of truth.
2. This reality is all pervading though intangible.
3. It is subjective and any attempt to describe it is at the cost of the reality. The revered Indian mystic Ramakrishna Paramhansa (1836–1886) put it beautifully: To attempt an intellectual understanding of such 'reality' is like a doll made of salt trying to measure the depth of sea.
4. In these conceptualizations, there is an emphasis on perception and that's it, rather than using it for volition or manipulation. Spiritual way of describing reality is full of paradox, is not falsifiable, and is nontangible.
5. These spiritual traditions prescribe the methods and tools to increase the capacity to perceive this kind of reality, though acknowledge the limitation of the individual in terms of their effort and capacity.
6. In spiritual endeavor, every time you start with the beginning. Unlike science which builds on itself and whatever is built is transferable to the next step, in spiritual work, one starts from scratch and reaches each time to one's own potential.

Now, the fact is that a core dualism exists in both western and eastern views of human existence. There is a dualism in both traditions of mind, i.e., western and eastern but the dualism fundamental to western thoughts is not similar to the dualism of Hindu thought. Descartes (1596–1650) most famously represents the western separation of the psychological self and the body as declares that while the self-thinks and lacks extension, the body is unthinking and extended. In other words, there are two types of realities in western dualism: (i) Physical reality, which is extended in space and empirically perceivable, and (ii) mental reality, which does not have spatial extension and is not empirically perceivable.

Hindu dualism differs from western dualism by regarding not just the physical body but also the mind, ego, thoughts, emotions, etc., belonging to the realm of inert matter. So in Hindu tradition dualism is not between the physical reality on one hand and mental reality on the other, but it is between pure awareness and all objects of awareness. Whether these objects are physical and extended or internal or nonextended. So thoughts, feelings, emotions, memory, etc., are as material or physical as the visible ingredient of the empirical world.

According to Hindu schema, pure consciousness called 'purusa' animates and pervades the mind, i.e., thoughts, emotion, craving but the two are completely distinct entities. There is thus a radical distinction between the mind, which is considered to be very subtle but nonetheless inanimate matter and pure consciousness which is the actual life force. Animated by the consciousness, it is the mind that imagines itself to be the real self rather than a material entity external to consciousness. The mind is therefore the seat of ignorance and bondage. Purusa is "witness, free, indifferent, a spectator and inactive". Therefore, the goal of all Indian liberation seeking thought in general is to extricate pure consciousness from its embroilment with the internal working of the mind as well as the external senses of the body.

Now if we extend this to the Buddhist way of thinking, which is a nondual system, in as sense that even notion of 'purusa'/pure consciousness is rejected. Consciousnesses is not an immutable and separate entity that can be uncoupled form the object of consciousness. Consciousness is ever-changing noneternal layer that exists only in interdependent relation to object of consciousness and not separate and autonomous from them. So the difference here in yoga is consciousness is separate from the object of consciousness and aim of life is to extricate itself from its enmeshment of the world. In contrast liberation in Buddhism, Nirvana is attained when one ceases to identify consciousness as eternal and unchanging and realizes that consciousness depends on object of consciousness and does not exist without this. Reality according to Buddha has three characteristics: (1) Annicha, everchanging. (2) Annata, impersonal, egoless, impersonal. (3) Dukkha, suffering.

I believe these are the very questions which psychoanalysis as a discipline has been trying to explore and trying to explain, mainly by investigating around 'ego'/ 'self'. I also see a kind of convergence (as well as difference) between psychoanalysis and spiritual/religious traditions. In spiritual traditions, self has been considered very much a problem, an illusion, ignorance and the approach is to transcendent it. Whereas in psychological or psychoanalytic it has been taken as a reality of its own accord. A 'reality' that needs to be adjusted with the 'reality' outside. Psychoanalytic approach is to modify 'I' and spiritual aspiration is to go beyond.

Krishnamurti and Bohm's collaborative work, *Ending of Time* (2014), brings this differentiation between 'chronological' and 'psychological time'. 'Personal or psychological time' and 'chronological and impersonal time'. Psychological time or personal time is time what is in our head, our personal concept of time. At simplistic level, my 1 hour is in my head or 1 hour according to me is not 1 hour according to this clock. The amount of time spent in so called '1 hour' by me, could be different for time spent in 1 hour by you. This personal/psychological kind of time has a quality of starting from somewhere, from a static point. And mostly it is related to 'me' or 'I'. So I call it personal time.

TOWARD SYNTHESIS AND CONCLUSION

Allow me now to offer a distillation of the ideas outlined above in a succinct manner. This consists of the following eight points:

1. A personal time starts with the origin of 'I.'
2. Personal time in terms of 'I' starts with my birth and finish with my death. It is different from time in a chronological sense, or in a sense of physics or impersonal time.
3. Unlike chronological time, this is absolute, has a definite start and definite end. On the other hand it does not move. I give an example. When I going to India recently, and I had a stop in Dubai. When I was in that transit, in terms of time I was thinking, few hours before I was in England, and after few hours I will be in India. Time in Dubai is 11 AM, time in UK at time was 8 AM and time in India should be 1:30 PM. In all these thoughts, there is this "I" is static and not moving and time is in relation to this 'I.' This fact becomes more obvious when you observe this whole phenomena from an impersonal view, like somebody else, who is observing, that this person of Nitesh was in England few hours ago, now is in UK, and next he will be in India. So this projection of time into the past or future is in relation to I, which is static.
4. The starting point of this personal time and I are same. This is from the act of first breath as this is the first act of volition, and a transition from being a passive recipient of life (where life was before being sustained by mother, through umbilicus) to an active seeker of life, and when this start it does not end till you die. In most of the ordinary circumstances, rest of the functions are taken care of by mother, breathing is something you have to take sole responsibility for. Mother cannot do it for the child.
5. 'I' is an inherent epiphenomenon in the act of volition. Simplistically when there is a stimulus, there is a response. This response is genesis of I, I who is separate from what I am acting upon. The only way I can explain this is. There is a famous quote by Archimedes pertaining to the lever mechanism, "give me the place to stand, and I shall move the Earth". So you need to be separate from who you are acting upon. So, observer is different from observation, because observer is observing. Seer is different from seen, because seer is seeing. Thought is different from the thinker, because thinker is thinking.
6. Across all organisms, this primitive I or act of volition is closely linked with the physical body and geared toward the act of self-preservation. Toward preserving life, and in systems language, keeping living system in ordered state at the expense of energy. Though reality is disorder will continue to increase, and this act of volition, and I will finish when life will finish.

7. In human being it seems, this I though is linked to the body, and that is the ultimate reality, but also gives appearance of being separate from the physical body. And having its own independence. An example of this is the phantom limb. Though the limb does not exist in real but one feels that one has a limb intact, one feel pain and all other sensation in that spatial dimension, where limb should have been present.
8. For me psychic reality involves relationship and movement between this 'I' and 'not I'. 'me' and 'not me'. Observer and observed. If I am still driving this 'Indian car' I mean car in my head (which is like motorbike) on British road, I am going to crash and if I am driving an English car (in my head) on Indian road, again I cannot drive.

By the relationship I mean a connection, an awareness of what is not me, and movement I mean able to get modified, change in response to 'not I'. In other words, we are in a continuous state where we are trying to match this personal/psychological time, with the chronological time, which is impermanent, ever changing, not absolute. Shaking the rigidity of personal time, and staying with the 'real' outside physical time in that sense. A spiritualist will say, aim to get rid of this psychological time/I, and then you do not need to adjust with real time all the time. You are physical time and with this ever-changing reality. Psychotherapist will say, let me offer you an observation and external reality and see if you can relate to that and not just that but also make that movement, which than changes everything around you. Or lets both of us or if we are in a group setting, all of us, try to align with this impersonal time, which is always in movement and change (and use each other as an anchor, support or that lever) and hope it moves our personal time not just in this session but outside this hour as well.

In order to link these observations with the psychoanalytic instinct theory, I will digress a bit and quote a passage from Freud's (1986) *An Outline of Psychoanalysis*.

> "After long hesitancies and vacillations we have decided to assume the existence of only two basic instincts, Eros and the destructive instinct (The contrast between the instincts of self-preservation and the preservation of the species, as well as the contrast between ego-love and object-love, falls within Eros). The aim of the first of these two instincts is to establish ever greater unities and to preserve them thus—in short, to bind together: The aim of the second is, on the contrary, to undo connections and so to destroy things. In the case of the destructive instincts we may suppose that its final aim is to lead living into an inorganic state. For this reason we also call it the death instinct. If we assume that living things came from inanimate ones and arose from them, then the death instincts fits in with the formula we have proposed

to the effect that instincts tend toward a return to an earlier state. In the case of Eros (or the love instinct) we cannot apply this formula. To do so would presuppose that living substance was once a unity which had later been torn apart and was now striving toward reunion" (p. 379–380).

His last two lines have a spiritual flavor and seem akin to the theological position which views human existence as having been being torn apart from God and eternally striving for a reunion with Him.[3] Given this all was alien to Freud's western mind, no wonder this aspect of his theory remained elusive and unclear.

I also do not agree that instinct of self-preservation and ego-love/object-love fall in the same category of Eros. Physical self and psychological self seems go in opposite direction. As I mentioned before, physical self or this physical body follow the rule of entropy, and chronological time. My view is ego, or as psychological-self does not. In fact I would say it is an obstacle to the reality outside. It does follow the rule of its own self-preservation, but that's the only rule it follow and at the expense of reality outside and this fear of annihilation, fuels its own life; even at the cost of physical life. Patrick De Mare (1991), a psychoanalyst and group analyst alludes to the same thing I am proposing that we 'death instinct' is nothing but is 'reality'. Which makes sense to me. Thenos is chronological time, a continuous movement toward disorder, i.e., entropy in terms of physics, and 'annicha' impermanence in Buddhist way. Pat De Mare proves this point when he says that psychical life seems to be more important than physical life which is evidenced by fact that people commit suicide to preserve this psychical life at the expense of physical life. Same way we can understand violence and homicide.

The above way of integrating psychoanalysis, group-dynamics and systems I presented in a talk (Painuly 2015) titled as 'Analysis through time' which essentially says the following:

- There is a divide between "observer" and "observed", me and not me, but as soon as we verbalize this concept it is in observation domain, not me. So there is no pure subjectivity. Observer is always included in the observation.
- Its obvious, observation depends on observer.
- As a concept, observer is a function of observation.
- For operational purposes 'personal me' is observer, which starts with birth (with the first act of violation, i.e., first breath) can be considered as a static observer, 'me'.

[3]Akhtar (2005) has made an attempt to link Freud's (1920) concept of death instinct with the eastern mystical tradition.

- Psychological/personal time start with the birth (with the origin of ego) and finishes with the death. In contrast to chronological time, personal time has a static reference point related to I and seems to have no movement which is inherent in chronological/impersonal time.
- Psychological self though start with the physical self, but at least in human being seem to run a kind of independent course of its own life (though in a false sense, as it cannot sustain it without physical life). This does not seem to follow the rule of reality in physical world, like irreversibility of time, law of entropy, etc.
- One of the way of understanding human struggle could be, a continuous effort to align this personal time with the outside, impersonal time which we can conceive as external reality. Spiritual aspirations are to get rid of this personal time. More modest approach is able to make it as flexible as changeable as chronological time through relationship, therapy, learning from experiences, etc. So commonality of minimizing this impact of psychological time as much as we can. Concept of mindfulness more or less says the same thing.
- Psychic reality involves movement and relationship between this very much divide of observation and observer, me and not me. Relationship I mean, an awareness or connection b/w 'me' and 'not me'. Movement I mean in different way, movement of time like chronological time, or the activity of modifying 'me' in view 'not me', which is impersonal.

Like the response to this talk, my ideas so far in therapeutic world were simply put as my fascination with 'primary narcissism'. I suppose there is an Indian in me who does not want to give up, as there is always that underlying knowledge deep inside we as humans are born with a sense of completeness and free of suffering, unlike psychoanalytic ideas where all we can do is to adjust with our suffering.

In my attempt to translate the different language (which as an immigrant you end up doing most of your life, translating for your therapist, for your patients, and later for your kids, etc.) the system as a whole could be translated as a 'self' as a whole, where all something which does not belong to me (not me) can be labeled as 'projected self' and what I call me or mine is 'identified self' and the split (something which has been be loosely translated as 'ignorance' and the driver of 'projective identification' and all its vicissitudes) which eventually belong to nothing but self as a whole (? Brahman).

Buddhist 'Nama-rupa' or Vedantic 'Maya' is probably similar to the way any system is defined 'i.e., anything which has a structure and function'. And systems-isomorphy (von-Bertalanffy, 1968) is not less a mystic principle which states all systems are similar in structure and function and are different in different context. In that regard the theory of living human system on which systems-centered work is based simply states 'a theory of living human system defines the hierarchy of isomorphic systems which are goal-directed, energy organizing and self-correcting' which in other words can be ascribed to anything which is called Maya in Indian spiritual tradition. Though these are just ideas or at best some tentative hypotheses. The real task is to develop some tangible and testifiable operational definitions and see if this all has any validity.

CODA

How do I make sense of my journey to become a 'medical psychotherapist' in a foreign land? I have no doubt that this journey was an attempt to work through something very personal and deep which has always been there troubling me but in India it was probably too close, enmeshed, and shielded by cultural defenses, that it was almost impossible to even see, let alone to be able to work on it. At the same time, I probably would have found some other way to work this through. There was also an attempt to make sense of the alienation of being in a different culture, and ability to grieve through the loss which is inevitable, so I can adjust in my 'new home' as best as possible. This probably created more valency for working in the group, where the culture itself becomes the explicit focus of investigation and also there is seduction and possibility of belonging in the group.

I cannot say I have achieved above tasks yet, but I like the idea of being in a journey rather than being 'stuck'. With time I have got better in tolerating the turbulence that we face when we are 'at the edge of the unknown'. I have developed more trust in the knowledge that any real change only happens when we cross this 'turbulence' and 'dread' with curiosity and compassion for oneself.

For last 3 years I have been working across two services namely Eating Disorders and Personality Disorders Service and given the different nature of both jobs where in Eating Disorders Service emphasis is more on my medical and psychiatric skills whereas in Personality Disorders Service I primarily work as a Medical Psychotherapist. There is no doubt managing these different roles at times is challenging but at the same time, I feel privileged that I have all these roles which all bring different resources available to help my patients and my team. I think I am beginning to integrate this internal split between 'either being a doctor or a therapist' in a more adaptive way.

From theoretical side, there are exciting developments happening in neuroscience, e.g., consciousness studies (Friston, 2010; Seth, 2021), polyvagal theory (Porges, 2011) and advances in theoretical physics (Penrose, 2005) which indicates reality is probably more on the side of the so called 'nondual'. Of-course, there is political and power dynamics in deciding which narratives are taken more seriously and are valued more, but my hunch is we as Indians do not need to rush to adapt the models which do not seem to fit our soul. I would prefer to find the opportunities where I can join 'similarities' whole heartedly and build it from there, and keep testing our assumptions and hypotheses in the true 'spirit' of science.

FURTHER READING

1. Agazarian YM, Gantt SP. Autobiography of a Theory: developing a theory of living human systems and its systems-centered practice. London: Jessica Kingsley; 2000.
2. Agazarian YM. Systems-Centered Therapy for Groups. New York: Guilford; 1997.
3. Agazarian YM. The visible and invisible group. London: Routledge; 1995.
4. Akhtar S. Freud along the Ganges: psychoanalytic reflections on the people and culture of India. New York: Other Press; 2005.
5. Balint M. The basic fault. London: Tavistock Publications; 1968.
6. Bertalanffy L. von General systems theory: Foundations, development, applications. New York, NY: George Braziller; 1968.
7. Clark DM. Implementing NICE guidelines for the psychological treatment of depression and anxiety disorders: The IAPT experience. Int Rev Psychiatry. 2011;23:375-84.
8. De Mare P, Piper R, Thompson S. Koinonia: from hate, through dialogue, to culture in the large group. London: Karnac; 1991.
9. Department of Health. New ways of working for psychiatrists: Enhancing effective, person-centred services through new ways of working in multidisciplinary and multi-agency contexts: Final report 'but not the end of the story'; 2005. [online] Available from https://core.ac.uk/download/pdf/97904.pdf [Last accessed December, 2023].
10. Foulkes SH, Anthony EJ. Group Psychotherapy: The Psychoanalytic Approach, 2nd edition. London: Pelican; 1965.
11. Freud S. Historical and expository work on psychoanalysis. Outline of psychoanalysis. The Pelican Freud Library. London: Pelican. 1986;15.
12. Friston C. The free energy principle: a unified brain theory? Nat Rev Neurosci. 2010;11(2):127-38.
13. Kakar S, Kakar K. The Indians: portrait of a people. New Delhi: Penguin; 2009.
14. Krishnamurti J, Bohm D. The ending of time: where philosophy and physics meet. New York, NY: HarperOne; 2014.
15. Lewin K. Field theory in social science. New York: Harper and Row; 1951.
16. Lewin K. Resolving social conflicts & Field Theory in Social Sciences. Washington, DC: American Psychological Association; 1997.
17. Little M. Winnicott working in areas where psychotic anxieties predominate: a personal record. Free Associations. 1985;3:9-42.
18. Mace C, Healy K. Medical psychotherapy: a specialty for now. The Psychiatrist. 2011;35:301-4.
19. Nitsun. The Anti-group: Destructive Forces in the Group and their Creative Potential. London: Rouledge; 1996.
20. Painuly N. A Letter from a Deviant. Systems-Centered News. 2020;28(2): 22.
21. Painuly N. A theory of living human systems (TLHS) and COVID-19. Systems-Centered News. 2020;28 (2):4-6.

22. Painuly N. Analysis through time. Guest lecture at Derbyshire Institute of Psychodynamic Psychotherapy. Derby, 6th May; 2015.
23. Painuly N. Case History submitted for PGDip in Psychodynamic Psychotherapy, University of Derby; 2009.
24. Painuly N. Critically examine the importance of dynamic administration in the setting up and maintenance of a therapeutic group culture. Theory essay submitted for Diploma in Groupwork Practice, Institute of Group Analysis, London; 2012.
25. Painuly N. My therapy through Yvonne's books. Systems-Centered News. 2021;29(2):29.
26. Painuly N. Projective identification in the spirit of 'join': elephant with no rider. Systems-Centered News. 2018;26(1):22.
27. Painuly N. Psychodynamic view of causality in human development: theory and practice. Submitted as a term paper for PGCert in Psychodynamic Psychotherapy, University of Derby; 2008.
28. Painuly N. Regression in therapy: some technical and therapeutic issues. Submitted as a term paper for PGDip in Psychodynamic Psychotherapy, University of Derby; 2009.
29. Painuly N. Re-viewing TLHS & its systems-centered practice through Kurt Lewin's legacy. Systems-Centred News. 2021;29 (1):9-16.
30. Painuly N. Using examples from clinical or other group situations, explore a group-analytic perspective on the impact of boundary breaches on the dynamics of the group. Reflective practice essay submitted for Diploma in Groupwork Practice, Institute of Group Analysis, London; 2013.
31. Penrose R. Shadow of the mind: a search for the missing science of consciousness. London: Vintage; 2005.
32. Porges SW. The polyvagal theory: neurophysiological foundations of emotions, attachment, communication, self-regulation. New York, NY: Norton; 2011.
33. Rosenfield H. Impasse and Interpretation: Therapeutic and Anti-therapeutic factors in the Psychoanalytic Treatment of Psychotic, Borderline and Neurotic patient. London: Routledge; 1987.
34. Seth A. Being you: a new science of consciousness. London: Faber & Faber; 2021.
35. Wakefield S, Kellett S, Melanie Simmonds-Buckley M, Stockton D, Bradbury A, Delgadillo J. Improving Access to Psychological Therapies (IAPT) in the United Kingdom: A systematic review and meta-analysis of 10-year of practice-based evidence. Br J Clin Psychol. 2021;60:1-37.

10

CHAPTER

Where in India is My Psychoanalytic Work?

Salman Akhtar

ABSTRACT

This contribution delineates the myriad ways in which the good aspects of Indian culture have become organized idioms of discourse for a US-based psychoanalyst of Indian origin. This impact is discernible in his theoretical formulations (especially his revision of Freud's death instinct concept and disdain of religious belief). It is also evident in his clinical praxis (through the subtly Indian decor of his office, the suffusion of 'Luckhnavi Tehzeeb' in his manner of relating, and the frequent appearance of Hindu mythology, Urdu poetry, and Bollywood songs in his counter-transference experience).

Keywords: India, Psychoanalysis, Culture, Death, Religion, Office, Therapeutic stance

INTRODUCTION

I met Masud Khan (1924–1989), the *enfant terrible* of psychoanalysis, 11 months before he died. The encounter, while informative, left me distressed and disillusioned. Here was a man ravaged by cancer, alcoholism, moral decay, and social ostracism. The contrast between the erudite psychoanalytic creator of concepts such as 'cumulative trauma,' 'symbiotic omnipotence,' and 'lying fallow' (Khan, 1963, 1969, 1983, respectively), and the bombastic, unkempt, and mad figure who was at one moment impishly charming and the next moment spewing anti-Semitic rants[1] was simply too great. Fortunately, this encounter occurred when I had already graduated from a psychoanalytic institute. This last point is important, for while 'growing up' as a psychoanalyst (a process which, as we all know, hardly stops with the formal end of analytic training and, in fact, might even begin at that point), I had made Khan as the object of 'forward projection of [my] narcissism' (Chasseguet-Smirgel, 1984). He hailed from my homeland, India[2], was a

[1]According to Paterson (1991), Khan's anti-Semitism was "peculiarly unconvincing" (p. 110). Two other British analysts, namely Baljeet Mehra and Charles Rycroft (quoted in Cooper, 1993), also suspected it to be an affectation. And, I have elsewhere (Akhtar, 2007) referred to it as a "band-aid of paranoid grandiosity" (p. 993) to keep a crumbling self-intact.

[2]Khan was born in British Imperial India and left the country for England before India was partitioned. So, by birth and formative upbringing, he was Indian, even though he later identified himself as Pakistani (since the region of his birth got included in the newly born nation).

fellow Muslim, an elegant writer, and, above all, renowned in the field of psychoanalysis. Being the only Indian candidate-in-training (1979–1987)[3], I desperately needed a homoethnic role model that could 'contain' (Bion, 1962) the nascent aspirations of my lonely, dark-skinned, Indo-Muslim, Urdu-speaking, psychoanalytic self. Having never met Khan in person sustained the idealization and by the time the hooked rope of my narcissistic climb broke, I had safely arrived on the roof, so to speak. The disillusionment hurt but did not break me; my developmental need of him had diminished by then.

The question, however, remains about the nature of this need. While excellent mentoring, sponsorship, and guidance (by Vamik Volkan, Selma Kramer, Otto Kernberg, Arnold Cooper, and Theodore Shapiro) had given me direction and strength, something deep in me was satisfied by my remote and imaginary Indo-Muslim connection with Khan. The only time I have been able to convey the ineffable yet profound nature of the loneliness that propelled my need for such a bond was when I once asked my distinguished colleague, Stanley Coen, the following question: "How would you feel if you were the only Jewish analyst in the world?" No more needs to be said, I think, on this matter.

It is with this internal position, split between a sense of belonging and a sense of aloneness in the field of psychoanalysis, that I began my professional journey. I became increasingly comfortable in my identity as a psychoanalyst as time passed but for decades remained uncertain about where did my ethnic, national, and ancestral roots fit in my analytic 'working ego' and 'working self' (Bolognini, 2008). The question that took hold of my system was this: Where is India in my psychoanalytic work? This paper is an attempt to document, categorize, and reflect upon the answers to this question that have appeared in my imagination and praxis over the nearly three decades of my postgraduate analytic career. I am aware that it is difficult to separate what is Indian in such insights and what is related to the specifics of my childhood. With this caveat, I will now present some areas of theory and practice that seem to have India's presence in them.

THEORY

I have tried to enrich two aspects of psychoanalytic theory by 'Indianizing' them. These include the controversial death instinct concept and the tedious impasse between psychoanalysis and religion. While I have decided to

[3]Fourteen years after my graduation, I learned that two individuals of Indian origin were also psychoanalytic trainees while I was a candidate. One was in Baltimore (Saida Koita), and the other in Michigan (Dushyant Trivedi). Both graduated from their respective institutes ahead of me (in 1981) but our paths did not cross till the year 2001.

focus upon these topics, there are other areas as well where I have tried to cross-fertilize Indian culture and psychoanalytic thought. These include the following:

- I have noted (Akhtar, 1999) that the degree of separation-individuation (Mahler et al., 1975) might be lesser in Indian children and the symbiotic phase might last much longer than it does in the West.
- I have agreed with Roland's (1998) proposal of a less differentiated 'we self' among Indians but with two caveats: The rural and urban Indians might defer in this regard *and* the 'we self' might co-exist with more individuated sectors of personality.
- I propose that the anal phase of psychosexual development is less repressed among Indians and its drive derivatives often contribute to pathological formations and clinical associations of Indian patients in analysis.
- I also believe that the degree of graphic imagery and the dramatis personae of the oedipal phase might differ in Indian and American childhood. Moreover, domestic servants can often play a significant role as 'containers' (Bion, 1962) of the erotic dimension of such triadic conflict.
- Finally, I hold that the back-and-forth movement between various levels of psychic maturity is greater among Indians. In my experience, young adults (and, even those more firmly established in adulthood) keep their child-like parts away from the gaze of their parents. They express such parts only with their partners, especially during play, sexual foreplay, and during vacations. Indian adults, however, tend to become regressed and can behave in a child-like fashion when visiting their parents. Far from being ego-threatening, such regression is mutually enjoyable and aims to restore the early parent-child bond, even though on a transient and illusory basis.

These passing, even if important, observations do not constitute the main modifications of psychoanalytic theory that I have attempted. They pertain to the concept of death instinct and the psychoanalytic perspective on religion. It is to these matters that I will now devote more sustained attention.

The Death Instinct

Based upon observations regarding children's turning traumatic experiences into play, certain analysands' returning over and over again to painful past experiences, the behavior of those who must go repeatedly through similar calamities, and the dreadful preoccupations of war veterans, Freud suggested that there might be a self-destructive "demonic force" (1920, p. 35) at work in them. This force worked in opposition to the pleasure principle and was aligned with a fundamental attribute of mind that searched for reduction of all excitation to quiescence. At its deepest, this search for quiescence—the 'Nirvana principle'—was aimed at returning the living organism to its previous, inorganic state. Freud (1920) thus gave voice to his celebrated though controversial concept of the 'death instinct'. A threat to the self at birth, this force is deflected outward by the influence of libido and ego using the agency of somatic musculature. Freud termed this outwardly deflected part of the death instinct the 'aggressive instinct'. In *The Ego and the Id* (1923), Freud added that the death instinct operates silently. In *Civilization and Its Discontents,* he emphasized that "aggressive instinct is the derivative and the main representative of the death instinct" (1930, p. 122). In *Analysis terminable and interminable* (1937), Freud referred to the death instinct and related masochism, negative therapeutic reaction, and unconscious guilt to this instinct's derivative: the aggressive drive. And, finally, in *An Outline of Psycho-analysis* (1938), he reiterated his formulation of "two basic instincts" (p. 148), one to establish unities and the other to undermine connections. He emphasized that the "concurrent and mutually opposing action of the two basic instincts gives rise to the whole variegation of the phenomena of life" (p. 149).

Freud acknowledged borrowing the expression 'Nirvana principle' from Barbara Low, a Sanskrit expert. The notion of 'death instinct', thus, from the beginning, had an Eastern touch. Gustav Fechner, the renowned physicist whose 'constancy principle' led Freud to the 'Nirvana principle', was himself involved in Buddhism (Jones, 1957). And, Romain Rolland, from whom Freud (1930) obtained the related concept of 'oceanic feeling', was an avid reader and biographer of the nineteenth-century Indian mystics, Sri Ramakrishna Paramahansa (1836–1886) and Swami Vivekananda (1863–1902). The Indian mystic tradition therefore seems to be a background conceptual source for Freud's death instinct. This might be a reason why the concept appeared alien to Western minds. With the exception of Klein (1933, 1935, 1952), her followers, and Eissler (1971), most subsequent analysts laid the postulate of death instinct to rest. In the Kleinian tradition, however, the concept remains, and it is utilized largely to explain mental operations that seek to destroy sublime thought, ego synthesis, and the capacity for in-depth object relations.

Subsequent elaborations by Rosenfeld (1971), Fayek (1980), Green (1999), Feldman (2000, 2009), Schmidt-Hellerau (2006) and Kernberg (2009) shared one thing in common: death instinct was invariably seen as something negative, problematic, and harmful to the mind. None of these analysts considered the possibility that the death instinct could serve as a loyal and reliable guide to our final destination. In contrast, I propose that the psychological repercussions of death instinct are not always distress-producing but can be the source of reassuring existential lullabies, especially towards the end of life. And, a close examination of psychoanalytic literature offers some support for my suggestion. It shows a recurring notion that there is, in humans, a vague, drive-like, internal pull towards the loss of the boundaries, if not the existence, of the psychic self. Concepts that allude to this internal pull include: (1) The merger fantasies, often associated with feeding and with sleep (Lewin, 1950); (2) the deep seated wish for loss of human identity by 'metamorphosis' (Lichtenstein, 1963); (3) the everlasting wish for "the lost, original union with the mother" (Jacobson, 1964, p. 39); (4) in the context of neonatal life, "the drive to return to an earlier state where all was gratified automatically" (Stone, 1971, p. 236); (5) man's eternal yearning to recapture the "co-anesthetically remembered harmony of dual-unity stage" (Mahler, 1971, p. 186); (6) the "search for oneness" (Kaplan, 1977); (7) man's "nostalgia for primary narcissism" (Chasseguet-Smirgel, 1984, p. 29), and (8) an attempted reconciliation of 'everything' and 'nothing' fantasies, which occurs "transiently in dreamless sleep and in the ecstasy of orgasm – but the promise of permanence can be realized only after our individual lives are over" (Shengold, 1991, p. 7).

To be sure, these concepts have diverse theoretical foundations, involve fantasy content not attributable to instinctual primitivity, and contain an unmistakable libidinal admixture with aggression. Yet, collectively, these notions demand contemporary reconceptualizations of the death instinct concept. Such examination might confirm the ubiquitous existence in humans of a deep-seated wish for the loss of self-boundaries, perhaps an echo of the primal desire for (and a dim memory of) merger with the mother. It might be that this preverbal pull subsequently accrues fantasies from various levels of psychosexual development. Death, too, may enter this scenario, though much after infancy and childhood, perhaps truly not even until middle age. From then onward, the deep-seated desire for fusion with mother might become intermingled with a longing for peace via death; thus, a 'death instinct' has been set into motion. Individuals who are traumatized by early losses through death or themselves have faced early life-threatening crises, might incorporate the notion of death into this substrate of fusion/oblivion seeking much earlier (Akhtar, 2001; Settlage, 2001). They might give evidence of their possessing a 'death instinct' even before middle age. Such a formulation of 'death instinct' is clearly different from the original one by Freud (1920).

In this reconceptualization, both words—*death* and *instinct*—appear misnomers. As one begins to digest this, another conundrum surfaces. This pertains to the fact that Freud often used the term 'death instinct' in its plural form. On at least eight occasions in *Beyond the Pleasure Principle* (1920: pp. 47, 49, 53 twice, 57, 60, 61, 63), in a letter to Max Eitingon (20 February 1920, cited in the Editor's Note to Freud's 1920 paper, p. 4), in *The Ego and the Id* (1923: pp. 46, 54, 59), in his succinct version of the libido theory (Freud,

1923, p. 258), and in *The Economic Problem of Masochism* (1924, p. 160), Freud talks of "death instincts" instead of "death instinct". This linguistic usage has received little attention, though it certainly appears curious. What could he have meant by 'death instincts'? Are there many types of them?

Having speculated on the various possible explanations of Freud's use of the plural 'death instincts' elsewhere (Akhtar, 2011a), I will focus here on the possibility that there are two types of death instinct. This can help explain the divergent perspectives on death itself: death as a threat to life versus death as a welcome relief from life. Here again, the West-East cultural difference comes into play. But matters are perhaps larger than that. The view of death as fundamentally unacceptable might be a manifestation of 'malignant' death instinct. The view of death as acceptable and, after a certain age, even desirable might be the product of 'benign' death instinct. The 'malignant' variety of death instinct might be responsible for attacks on linking, black holes in the mind, autoimmune disorders, and intense sadomasochism. The 'benign' variety of death instinct might be responsible for positive emptiness, dreamless sleep, fallow states of mind, and the psychic pause that often precedes a creative act. If the distinction along these lines holds, then the phenomenological scene involving the two death instincts would appear quite different. It would be evident that the 'malignant' variety marches on the drumbeat of impending self-implosion while the 'benign' variety sings soothing lullabies for eternal rest.

Enter Mirza Asad-Ullah Khan Ghalib (1797–1869). The mid-nineteenth century doyen of Urdu poetry in India was "one of the greatest poets South Asia has ever produced", according to the Oxford University scholar, Ralph Russell (2000, p. 8). Ghalib took the stance that death is *a part* of life and not *apart* from life. Far from providing a container of morbid projections, his viewpoint—containing echoes of advaitic Hindu mysticism (Vallabhneni, 2005) and the Sufi tradition of Islam (Shafii, 2008)—regards death as a liberating union (re-union?) with the cosmos-at-large and a great sense of freedom by the renunciation of self. Freud's (1920) grim declaration that "the aim of all life is death" (p. 38) was long preceded by Ghalib's (1841) lyrical pronouncement that *"Ishrat-e-qatra hai dariya meiN fana ho joana"* (literally: "it is pure ecstasy for a rain-drop to fall upon a river and lose itself altogether").[4] Consider also the following couplet by Ghalib:

"Ghum-e-hasti ka Asad kis se ho juz marg ilaaj
Shamma hur rung mein jalti hai sahar hone tak" (p. 31).

---

[4]Such literal translation of this line (and of all other Urdu verses that follow) invariably result in a regrettable loss of prosodic beauty and kindling potential of the words chosen by the poet. I therefore feel sorry for all three parties involved here—the poet, myself as an amateur translator, and the reader—for this loss.

Literally translated, this couplet means that just the way the beginning sunlight at the time of dawn relieves the candle from the continued necessity to burn, the arrival of death cures all problems of life. Let me cite another of Ghalib's (1841) couplets.

> "*Partav-e-khur se hai shabnam ko fanaa ki taleem*
> *Main bhi hoon, ek inaayat ki nazar hone tak*" (p. 60).

This one, in literal translation, means that just the way warm rays of sun teach the dew drops the art of vanishing, one kind glance of the Creator will readily draw me back to Him; I exist only till that graceful moment arrives.

Of note in these two examples (and I could have given many others) are the following elements: (i) Death is recognized to be a natural and expectable event without which life remains incomplete; (ii) the attitude towards death is neither ostrich-like denial nor masochistic celebration but total acceptance, and, (iii) an admixture of relief and sacred joy is also seen to be associated with the experience of death. The metaphors utilized by Ghalib (e.g., 'drop-river merger', 'sunshine-dew drop connection', 'the candle's having to burn till morning') subtly but unmistakably pronounce death to be a merger with something larger than oneself, a return and fusion with the cosmos at large. The accompanying loss of self is implied to be a pleasant, even ecstatic occurrence.

This is certainly different from Freud's (1926) *Todesangst*. In all fairness, however, it must be acknowledged that Freud took both positions, i.e., death is something to be feared, despised, and regarded as an enemy of life (1923, 1926) and, death is something to be accepted, patiently waited for, and even joyously welcomed for offering us relief from the internal and external conflicts that characterize life (1920, 1937). As a result, what appears to be a tension between Ghalib and Freud also reflects the tension between the contradictory views of Freud himself. Study of Indian mysticism and Urdu poetry thus helps unmask this conceptual bifurcation in Freud's theorizing.

Religion

By the very act of making God a subject of metapsychological deconstruction, Freud took a resolutely atheistic position. His pupils and followers adhered 'religiously' to the arguments and declarations he made in *The Future of An Illusion* (Freud, 1927) and later in *Civilization and Its Discontents* (1930). Scientific positivism of the early twentieth century provided a receptive crucible for Freud's debunking of God. He had given voice to what was brewing in the minds of the Western intelligentsia. The unspeakable atrocities that soon followed in the name of religious nationalism in Europe 'confirmed' that ethnocentrism and religious belief were dangerous commodities. They led to intoxication with in-group superiority and laid the groundwork for oppression of 'others', and even cruelty and genocide. Early European psychoanalysts, themselves the victims of prejudice and violence, wholeheartedly followed the ray of hope offered by Freud's declaration that religion was a hoax and science will sooner or later assure that rationality prevails in the conduct of interpersonal and communal affairs. Atheism and psychoanalysis became inseparable.

The focus on the content of the *Illusion* book, however, distracted attention from its form which had the interesting feature of a dialogue with a conceptual opponent. To be sure, Freud had used this literary device elsewhere (e.g., 1915–1916) as well, but never with the ferocity as in his book on religion. The exchange between Freud and his imaginary, God-believing interlocutor fills the pages of *The Future of an Illusion*. But who actually is this religious 'friend' of Freud's? Think for a minute. What conclusion would a practicing analyst draw upon encountering an analysand who constantly talks of a friend with an opinion opposite to him? For instance, what would one think of a philanthropist on the couch who talks incessantly about a selfish and miserly friend of his? Or, of a shy academic who does not tire of mocking his exhibitionistic colleagues? What do their preoccupations betray? Now apply the answer to the debate between the self-declared 'Godless Jew' and his 'religious interlocutor' and you will arrive at the following conclusion: Freud was arguing with himself. Sheldon Bach's (1977) proposal that a split-off sector of the self invariably shows a 'mirror complementarity' with conscious protestations of the individual speaks to this very point. Let me put it bluntly: The '*Illusion*' monograph is a literary battlefield where 'Freud, the Atheist' is involved in a bloody combat with 'Freud, the Believer'!

This makes Freud all too human in my opinion. After all, struggles between theism and atheism are as psychically ubiquitous as the struggles between activity and passivity, spontaneity and restraint, homosexuality and heterosexuality, morality and immorality, and, above all, between living and dying. The debate about God's existence is hardly alien or new. It has raged on throughout mankind's history and impressive proponents of both sides in this choice are found in Greek and Roman civilizations. Even the Hindus, who are naively portrayed in the West as a God believing demographic monolith, have had a tradition of arguing about the existence of God that goes back at least to 2000 years before the birth of Christ (Sen, 2005).

With this in mind, Freud appears hardly peculiar for being conflicted about believing (or not believing) in God. It was his keeping the two sides of his ambivalence rigidly apart and professing conscious allegiance to only one side (while the other side the lurked just beneath the surface) that makes him interesting. His '*Illusion*' book is arresting due to the very tension of such ambivalence. And, frankly, the same conflict is evident in Freud's personal correspondence. He emphatically declares himself to be an atheist at one place and professes gratitude to God at another. The examples of the former include "I am a God-forsaken incredulous Jew" (letter to James Putnam, quoted in Nicholi, 2002, p. 63), "Neither in my private life nor in my writings I have ever made a secret of being an out and out unbeliever" (letter to Charles Singer, quoted in Gay, 1988), and "Why did none of the devout create psychoanalysis? Why did one of have to wait for a completely Godless Jew?" (letter to Oscar Pfister, quoted in Gay, 1988). Compare this with what Armand Nicholi, Jr. tells us in his book *The Question of God* (2002):

> "Letters throughout Freud's life are replete with words and phrases such as 'I passed my examinations with God's help'; 'if God so wills'; 'the good Lord'; 'taking the Lord to task'; 'into the keeping of the Lord'; 'until after the Resurrection'; 'science seems to demand the existence of God'; 'God's judgment'; 'God's will'; 'God's grace'; 'God above'; 'if someday we meet above'; 'in the next world'; 'my secret prayer'. In a letter to Oscar Pfister, Freud writes that Pfister was 'a true servant of God' and was 'in the fortunate position to lead others to God'" (p. 51).

Freud's comment upon meeting the Nobel Prize-winning Indian poet, Rabindranath Tagore (1861–1941), that "he really looks like what we imagine the Lord God looks like" (cited in Goldman, 1985, p. 293) is a similar testimony to his constant preconscious dwelling upon the subject of God. Now, it can be asserted that such references to God are not to be taken seriously. They are merely metaphorical and reflect nothing but a manner of speech and a touching affectation. But *that* is precisely my point—namely, that Freud had two pictures of God in mind. One was an anthropomorphized, concrete, and stern but protective Father-like presence which he resolutely defied. The other was a sublime object of wonder, humility, and gratitude to which he gladly paid homage. The former demanded idolatry which revolted Freud. The latter evoked humility, which Freud was fearless to experience.

Freud's first God is 'up there' and his second God is 'everywhere'. This tension becomes more evident if we bring in Wilfred Bion's (1965) concept of 'O' to bear upon the debate. I have elsewhere (Akhtar, 2009a) summarized what Bion meant by 'O' in the following passage:

> "Term used by Wilfred Bion (1965, 1967, 1970) to denote the ultimate truth of the moment or for the thing-in-itself, which is immeasurable. This truth is out there, waiting to be found by a receptive mind that has emptied itself of preconception, memory, and desire. Acquired knowledge can prepare the platform from which the leap of faith is taken, but it is leaving knowledge and experience behind that actually constitutes a step toward 'O'. Take, for instance, the Oedipus complex, or, for that matter, the mathematical equation, $E = mc^2$; these truths existed

long before 'Sophocles,' Sigmund Freud's and Albert Einstein's discovery of them. In other words, 'O' is the absolute truth and the supreme godhead of pure veracity" (p. 192).

Applied to the idea of ever-present Truth as God itself (or, at least, what I have called here Freud's 'second God'), we begin to note that Freud's God is sculpted in human terms. Bion's God is painted in the watercolor of wisdom. Freud's God is that of Judeo-Christian and Islamic traditions. Bion's God represents advaitic Vedantism, which is an antecedent of the modern Hinduism and Zen Buddhism (Vallabhneni, 2005). Freud's God speaks to the selected few. Bion's God sings through the murmur of the wind and floats on the waves of rivers and oceans. Freud's God can be accepted or refuted, Bion's God is inescapable.

But wait. Didn't I conclude that Freud had two versions of God in mind, one which he rebelled against in the '*Illusion*' book and the other that he thanked profusely in his private correspondence? One way to solve this conundrum is to equate 'Freud's God' and 'Bion's God' in the preceding paragraph with these two views held by Freud himself.

Even more interesting is that while neither Freud nor Bion mention woman/mother in connection with the origins of God, the foundation of their ideas seems to be in their early mothering experience and its rupture. Freud's traumatic loss of a beloved Catholic nurse maid (who frequently took him to church and in whose emulation he, as a child, preached to everyone) led to his massive repudiation of religion and music, the two phenomena associated with her memory. Bion's traumatic separation from the Hindu *Aaya* (nanny) of his childhood in rural India[5] led to the split result that he never traveled back to India but incorporated the Sanskrit word *Om* for the Omnipresent Creator in an abbreviated form 'O' (deleting the labial consonant 'm' that requires closing the mouth and ending the sound; both these actions are emblematic of separation) and described ideas about faith (see also Eigen, 1981; Neri, 2005) that have an unmistakable Eastern ring to them.[6] Both Freud and Bion were responding, albeit in a starkly different manner, to their early 'maternal' losses in formulating their ideas about faith and transformative higher powers.

A further proposal I have is this. Because both Freud and Bion had heteroreligious introjects (Freud, a Jewish child with Christian God within,

[5]A movie on Bion's life (which mostly for financial reasons remained unfinished) produced by the British group therapist, Meg Harris, depicts the tender mythological base of the Hindu nanny's dialogue with little Wilfred.

[6]Bion's pre-eminent exponent, Rafael Lopez-Corvo (2003), has also concluded that the concept of 'O' comes from India. Lopez-Corvo also provides other instances of Bion's memories of India and implies their impact upon his theorizing.

and Bion, a Christian child with Hindu God within), psychoanalysis could not comfortably accept religion. Freud's split with Jung, who was far more favorable to spirituality and mysticism, also resulted in firming up the analysis-religion antipathy. Far different from this was the situation of British Anglo-Saxon analysts, such as WRD Fairbairn, Donald Winnicott, and Harry Guntrip, who belonged to the ethnic majority in their country, did not encounter prejudice, and in fact had considerable religious education. They comfortably practiced their religion and even imbued their theories with it. Winnicott's (1962) concept of the 'survival of the object', for instance, has an undeniable resemblance to the resurrection of Christ.[7]

All in all, it seems that if the Judeo-Christian and Islamic views of God are tempered by the Hindu-advaitic view of God (Vallabhneni, 2005) and by the transference containing functions of Hindu deities (Rao, 2005; Kakar, 2007), then the question of God's existence becomes one that is actually not to be asked. God seems then to belong—like play and creativity—to the realm of the 'intermediate area of experience' (Winnicott, 1953). Such 'Indianization' softens the psychoanalytic viewpoint on God and expands the scope of theory and clinical praxis alike.[8]

PRACTICE

In discussing the suffusion of India in my clinical work, I will divide my comments into categories that pertain to my: (i) Office décor, (ii) mother-tongue, (iii) therapeutic attitude, and (iv) analytic technique.

Office Decor

In a detailed elucidation of the significance of the analyst's office for the analyst, analysand, analytic process, and analytic technique (Akhtar, 2009b), I emphasized that the office must be comfortable and kept consistent. Moreover, in setting the office up, one must avoid ostentatiousness as well as undue self-effacement. Both can make the office 'too noticeable' and impede its 'holding' (Winnicott, 1960) functions. I also noted that even more important is the feature of authenticity. This has to be achieved without undue self-disclosure. Thus, a painting that one is truly fond of, knick-knacks bought during one's travels, little statues and mementos given by loved ones belong in the office, whereas family photographs do not. Professional

[7]The recent book by Marie Hoffman (2000) titled, *Toward Mutual Recognition: Relational Psychoanalysis and the Christian Narrative*, contains many illustrations of this sort.

[8]Three books that I have edited (Akhtar, 2001, 2005; Akhtar and O'Neil, 2011) contain more details on this topic. What I wish to emphasize here is that I made sure that an India-Hindu perspective was included in all three works.

diplomas and awards fall somewhere between these two categories. The main point is to protect the analytic office from 'over-personalization' (Kersun and Silberman, 2005) and yet offer a blend of personal and professional ambience. It should be remembered that "the consulting room represents the interior of the object for which the analyst stands, filled with various part objects. In unconscious phantasy, all the concrete objects to be seen form parts of the analyst" (Carpelan, 1981, p. 153).

While Carpelan's statement referred mostly to the unconscious phantasy of the analysand, it is equally applicable, I think, to the analyst. After all, the analyst's cultural-aesthetic-and moral compass inevitably contributes to his or her office décor. If thus so, the question arises 'where is India in my office?' And, the answer is that it is present in the form of the following accoutrements (i) Two little statues of Ganesha, the elephant-headed Hindu deity and, (ii) a large painting which contains a quatrain by the renowned Urdu poet, Faiz Ahmad Faiz (1911–1984).[9] These two items are cultural icons that anchor my Indo-Muslim self. Ganesha is the Lord of Auspicious Beginnings for Hindus but it signifies something different for me. Besides reminding me of India in general, it signifies the fumbling clumsiness of compromise formation and the inevitable need to re-work decisions made in a hurry. After all, Ganesha acquired his elephant head after being beheaded as a human child by his father, Lord Shiva, who was furious when the boy stopped him (without knowing that Shiva was his father) from entering the private chambers of his mother (and Shiva's consort) Parvati. Once Shiva realized that he had caused immense distress to her, he immediately replaced the boy's decapitated head with that of the first animal he could find (an elephant). However, the mythmakers of India placed an elephant in Shiva's sight (and not a tiger, bear, or goat) because that animal, in India, is known for his long-term memory. In essence, the fable conveys two points: (i) Compromise formations are never fully satisfactory and, (ii) decisions arising out of 'manic defense' (Klein, 1935) will retain unconscious memory of their inherent incompleteness and therefore would need to be worked through later. The two Ganeshas in my office are thus sources of both impetus and solace in the protracted work of psychoanalysis. Why two? one might ask. This is a legitimate question and the best I can say is that my brother and I are the only children of our parents and most likely the two Ganeshas reflect this feature of the family iconography.[10]

---

[9]Like Masud Khan, Faiz Ahmad Faiz was born in undivided India and was thirty-six when the country got partitioned. Though he later identified himself as Pakistani, in my eyes, he remained Indian.

[10]Clearly, these reconstructions are the product of self-analytic work done in the course of writing this paper. The choice of the physical objects described here was, at the time of its execution, purely aesthetic.

The painting that contains a quatrain by Faiz Ahmad Faiz (1952) has its own 'holding' function. The poem reads:

> *Na pooch tub se tera intezaar Kitna hai*
> *Ki jin dinoN se mujhe tera intezaar nahiN*
> *Tera hi aks hai in ajnabi bahaaroN meiN*
> *Jo tere lub, tere abroo, tera kinaar nahiN*
> (p. 70)

Literally translated, the four lines mean:

> Don't ask, please, how desperately I have waited for you
> From the days, especially, when I gave up waiting for you
> Each facet of this oncoming spring reflects you
> Though none of them match, your lips, your eyebrows,
> your warm embrace

Now, the poem has a threefold emotional significance for me. One, it connects me with my mother-tongue, Urdu, and, by extension, to my mother and my motherland. Two, since my father, the renowned Urdu poet, Jan Nisar Akhtar (1914–1976), was a friend of Faiz Ahmad Faiz, the framed poem links me with my father. The coexistence of such links with mother and father, in turn lays down the oedipal foundation of the clinical space. And finally, by extolling the virtue of waiting and linking the manifest with the dormant, the poem celebrates the long and slow-moving psychoanalytic process itself. Coltart's (1986) celebrated essay, *Slouching towards Bethlehem*, comes to mind in this context and especially the passage where Coltart says that "the necessity of retaining faith in the analytic process, the outcome of which can never be foreseen, which in turn depends on the capacity to wait—without closing down by premature interpretation—for the 'rough beast' that is struggling to be born in the patient" (p. 102).

Mother-tongue

The occasional desire of the immigrant analyst to intervene in his mother-tongue (which the patient does not understand) usually has to be met with ego restraint and further grief work regarding the analyst's own immigration.[11] What is also needed at such moments is self-analytic inquiry into the specific transaction that triggered such a wish. In other words, the analyst must ask himself the following questions: What was in the patient communication that made me want to respond in my mother-tongue? Did the patient's

[11] In a sad commentary upon the long-lasting effects of Western colonialism, analysts from the third world countries seem to experience a greater reluctance about speaking in their respective mother-tongues.

words or feelings touch something deeply personal in me? What? And—in a return to a more objective stance—would it be useful to say the idea in my mother-tongue and then translate it for the patient? Or, should I just offer a translation? What is the advantage of the former? What would be lost by taking the latter route? Would speaking in my mother-tongue traumatize the patient or impart genuineness to the relational matrix?

These dilemmas are especially powerful for me since I grew up in a highly literary family (with seven generations of renowned literary scholars and poets on my father's side) and had parents who were devoted to writing (father a great poet, mother a distinguished literary critic and letter-writer of fame). My mother-tongue is very, very important to me. As a result, clinical dilemmas involving the use or nonuse of it have special significance for me. To illustrate this dimension of my clinical experience, I offer the following clinical vignettes:

Clinical Vignette 1

Dr Suzanne Berkeley,[12] a young internist, was looking after a hospitalized old man. Both of them were avid gardeners and often exchanged notes about their hobby with each other. In her analysis, one day she told me that the old man had given her some seeds that she was planning to plant in her backyard over the weekend. She was excited since the seeds were for a very rare type of flowering plant. "Old man", "backyard", "seed", and "flower" clearly constituted thinly veiled allusions to an oedipal transference fantasy. However, more important for the context, here is what happened the next day.

Suzanne began sobbing as soon as she entered my office. Her patient had died the previous night. She cried and said, "What good are those seeds now? I can't tell him how they fared. Did the flowers come out or not? It's all useless now. I'm just going to throw the seeds away." Listening to this, I was moved. The urge to say the following in Urdu came over me: *"Sub kahan, kuch laala-o-gul mein numayan ho gayeen."* The line from Ghalib (1841), is one of the two constituting the couplet:

> *Sub kahaN, khuch laala-o-gul meiN numayaN ho gayeeN.*
> *Khaak meiN kya soorateN hongi, jo pinhaN ho gayeeN* (p. 90).

Roughly translated, these lines mean: 'Not all, only a few of the buried ones emerge as flowers: The Earth's bosom hides so many faces, talents, and powers'. Given my cultural background of an ethnic and familiar

[12]The names given to patients in this paper are all fictitious. Also, I would like to acknowledge that some of these vignettes have appeared in my prior writings (Akhtar, 2009b, 2011, 2013).

tradition of offering rejoinders in the form of a single line of famous poem, it was the perfect empathic remark to make.[13] It would have conveyed to the listener that I resonated with her pain, helplessness, and sense of loss. However, in the clinical situation, where the patient did not understand my mother-tongue, I chose not to speak the words that had come spontaneously to my mind. I realized that uttering those words and then translating them would shift her attention from felt pain to intellectual effort; hearing me speak in a different language might disturb her.[14] A comment intended to be empathic with her mourning would become just the opposite for me (i.e., a manic defense) and a distraction for her. So I did not say it. However, in not saying it, I tolerated the helplessness of her not being linguistically receptive to me (like the old man was not available to her in reality anymore!). Like her, I also experienced a loss.

At another time, however, I did speak in my mother-tongue, Urdu, to a patient who, while multilingual, did not know that particular language.

Clinical Vignette 2

Naomi Jacobs was an intelligent and successful woman in her thirties. Her parents had become divorced when she was 7-year-old though she had sensed her father's increasing remoteness for a year or two before that. Following the divorce, Naomi felt 'invisible' to her father, who paid much more attention to her older sister and brother. The theme of her 'invisibility' came up frequently in her analysis and was found to be linked, at its base, to an early maternal depression and a pervasive maternal tendency to invalidate her feelings. It was also related to her father's lack of interest as well as her own defensive retreat from being 'visible' to him, since that stirred up all kinds of longings and desires. We worked this through and the patient established a solid romantic partnership with a man. One day she asked me what the word for 'daughter' in my mother tongue. I responded by saying that I was

---

[13]Upon hearing this vignette, a prominent New York analyst said that the idea of reciting poetry in a psychoanalytic session would appear pompous and exhibitionistic to him. The difference in the intellectual and aesthetic traditions that formed our childhood and our psychostructural backgrounds might account for the difference in what, stylistically, is permissive within our analytic work egos.

[14]During a post-termination contact, some 5 years later, I shared this dilemma with the patient; this time I did utter the words that had been in my mind in Urdu many years ago. I asked her how she might have responded had I spoken to her in my mother-tongue during that particular session. The patient, who had little memory of it, said that she would have been shocked. It was her sense that my decision to not speak to her in my mother-tongue at that time was most likely correct.

curious about what lay behind her question. Fantasies about my having a daughter emerged. Naomi expressed curiously about how I treated my daughter: better than her father treated her or the same way? Work along these lines led to further oedipal transference material as well as issues of sibling rivalry (her older sister had been the father's favorite).

However, when in a similar session a few days later she again asked me the Urdu word for 'daughter', I responded by saying "I guess you want to hear the word *beti* from me not only to satisfy your intellectual curiosity but to see with what feeling tone I utter it and also so that I can say it not only in front of you, but as if *to* you." Naomi nodded and began sobbing. I knew that I could have made the same interpretation without the use of the Urdu word *beti*, but felt that hearing it would provide just the right amount of gratification to her against which further mourning of her father's inattention towards her (and her anger about this) could take place. I am aware that some colleagues would argue that this gratification bypassed the analysis of her aggression. I do not agree with that view as there were plenty of other occasions for her discharging and analyzing aggression and because I believe that good analytic technique needs optimal and not maximal frustration in order for the patient to remain in an analyzable mode.

Unlike this example, uttering the Urdu word for the female genital during the analysis of an Indian woman posed a different sort of challenge for me. The hurdle I had to cross was not only technical but also tested the limits of my moral and aesthetic Indian idiom of life.

Clinical Vignette 3

A 50-year-old Hindu Indian woman, Sunita Jha, had been raised by an instinctually repressed (and repressive) family in South Africa, and spoke mainly in English during her analysis. As early fears of criticism and rejection were interpretively softened, a devalued self-image emerged. While childhood experiences of prejudice due to skin color were emphasized at first, analysis gradually revealed profound rejection by her mother, a rejection centering upon her being female. Work along these lines relaxed her further and occasionally began to speak in Hindi, her mother tongue. During one such session, Sunita very hesitantly revealed that she did not know the word for the female genital in Hindi and felt that it would help her to acquire this knowledge. Issues of maternal transference (i.e., can I label her body parts for her?; do I know and accept that she has female genitalia?; do I accept "my" female genitalia?, etc.) were clearly evident and I handled them in the customary analytic fashion.

However, in a later session, she quite earnestly asked me to tell her the word. Suddenly, I found myself experiencing a dual dilemma. One was a purely technical dilemma, i.e., what would be the process-related pros and cons of telling her the word as against inquiring as to why she wanted to know it from me, and so on. The other dilemma which caught me by surprise involved my personal morality, as it were. Can I even utter the word in my mother-tongue (spoken Hindi and Urdu have the same word for the female genital) in the presence of a woman? Experiencing the inhibition outlined nearly a century ago by Ferenczi (1911), for a moment, I became tongue-tied.[15] Then working through the inner block and in the spirit of "developmental work" (Pine, 1997) that includes occasionally providing patients with words for what is hard for them to express, I decided to tell her that it was called *choot*. I was aware of the potential transference gratifications in this intervention but the subsequent flow of our work confirmed my hunch that letting her hear the word from me would facilitate and not impede our access to that material.

In contrast to the two situations where I deliberately chose to use a particular word from my mother tongue and that, too, in response to the patient's request, the following vignette shows a spontaneous and deeply affectionate recitation of two lines of Urdu poetry as an 'affirmative intervention' (Killingmo, 1989) with a patient who, curiously, did not know the language at all.

Clinical Vignette 4

Katherine O'Malley had lost her mother to lung cancer at the age of four and a half. Although her father was very loving, her stepmother's duty-bound, anti-instinctual, and humorless attitude left Katherine with a life-long wound of maternal loss. She achieved great success in her profession, married, and raised two kids but always felt that something was missing from her life; a gnawing anguish persisted. This became worse when her teenage daughter got into drugs. Katherine now entered analysis and was surprised to discover the pervasive, even if subtle, effects of the childhood maternal loss upon her psychosocial

[15] A few years ago, a young Iranian candidate said to me: "I will die if I have to say the words for sex and genitals in Persian to a patient": (personal communication, April, 11, 2001, name withheld upon request). I smiled and encouraged her to explore this issue further on her own as well as in her analysis. I also reassured her that she was not alone in experiencing such anxieties, adding that even Freud lapsed into the Latin *matrem nudam* while describing, at age 41, the childhood memory of having seen his mother naked (letter to Fliess, October 3, 1897, in Masson, 1985, p. 268).

functioning. Grieving that had been 'deferred' (Freud, 1918) now began in earnest and occupied center stage for the first 2 years of her analysis.

In the fourth year, when such mourning seemed to have subsided, a disturbing external event re-kindled the grief. Katherine was overwhelmed and began crying profusely during one session. Barely able to stop heaving and sobbing, she said, "I thought it was over but surely, it is not". I felt moved to respond and said, "You know, two lines from a poem in my mother-tongue came to mind in response to what you just said. I know you will not understand them but let me recite them first and then I will translate them for you". After this, I recited, "*Kitne toofaN uthhaye aankhoN ne // Naao yaadoN ki doobti hi nahiN //*[16] I then paused and said, "It means that how many, just how many storms my eyes have borne but this goddamn boat of memory never sinks". Feeling understood and well 'held', Katherine nodded and became calmer.

What would have happened had I only offered the translated version? What was gained by my speaking in Urdu (knowing that Katherine did not understand it)? And, what would have been lost by not speaking in Urdu? Certainly since points can be debated *ad nauseum* but my clinical sense was that in speaking Urdu, I would not distract her too much and that by offering something of my mother-tongue (my mother), I was putting a sonorous salve over her wound of loss. I was also showing her that her experience had affected me deeply and this brought us closer. Finally, by putting her pain into words, I was helping her mentalize it and by presenting the pain of loss in a foreign language, I was universalizing and humanizing it.

This vignette and the two preceding it show the restraint (clinical vignette 1), selective and deliberate use (clinical vignettes 2 and 3), and spontaneous and affirmative offering (clinical vignette 4) of an immigrant analyst's mother-tongue. At times, however, the psychic activity encoded in one's mother-tongue is far more subtle and appears only in the form one's adopted, second language takes.

Clinical Vignette 5

Sy Goldman, a highly successful lawyer in his early 40's, had entered analysis soon after he was passed over for promotion in his law firm. A charming, well-spoken, well-dressed, and well-mannered man, Sy nonetheless suffered from deep insecurities about himself. One aspect of it pertained to his being a Jew; he was embarrassed about it and put forth every effort to 'hide' his ethnicity and to 'pass' as a Gentile.

[16]The line comes from a poem by the contemporary Urdu poet of India, Akhlaq Mohammad Khan Shahryar (1936–2012).

As analysis progressed, we traced the origin of this self-loathing to orally-determined greed (largely for sex) and resulting inner-shame and guilt over it. Sy had been raised by an accomplished but cold mother and an ineffective, castrated father. His hunger grew over his formative years, turned into greed and, in turn, led to inner-shame.

As all this was worked through, Sy became more comfortable with his ethnic identity. He joined a synagogue. And, just about then, he 'accidentally' found out that I was Muslim. He felt very ashamed of that and had great difficulty telling me that. When he did reveal it to me, I said, "You know, you have been ashamed of your being a Jew, and now you are ashamed of my being a Muslim. I think we need to explore how these two shames are related to each other. I paused for a moment and then added, "Are they sisters?"

Now, the addition of the last phrase was logically unnecessary, since the point had been made. The reflexive spurt from my unconscious therefore reflected something else, something poetic. And, why 'sisters'? (And not 'brothers'?). As I reflected upon this linguistic choice later, it became evident to me that in linking his two 'shames' as siblings, I was emphasizing the kinship of blood between my patient's 'owned' and 'projected' self-devaluation. But the word 'sisters' itself emanated from the fact that the Urdu words for shame and shyness (*sharm* and *haya*) are gendered as feminine!

Unlike this 'unmentalized' contribution of my mother-tongue to an interpretation, there are 'unspoken' contributions of my mother-tongue that facilitate receptivity to the clinical material being offered.

Clinical Vignette 6

In one of her turmoil-ridden analyses, Josephine Heller, a 40-year-old research scientist, told me of a ruthless and rather cruel berating by her husband. The details she laid out are chilling. However, it was when she ruefully added that once he seemed certain of having devastated her, he started to act very gentle and kind towards her. She could, however, discern the patronizing contempt in such 'love'. As she was talking, I found myself inwardly repeating a line from Ghalib: "*Ki mere qatal ke baad, us ne jafaa sey toba*" (literally: after killing me, he decided to renounce cruelty forever). My 'listening' to her in my mother tongue signaled that something usually deep was at work between us.

The boundary between empathy and countertransference becomes blurred under such circumstances. I will return to this point via Clinical Vignette 11 (see below).

Therapeutic Attitude

Elsewhere (Akhtar, 2009b), I have delineated three fundamental aspects of a positive therapeutic attitude: survival, vision, and faith. *Survival* (Winnicott, 1968) refers to the analyst's capacity to withstand erotic seductions and sadomasochistic assaults upon his work ego and steadfastly maintain his analytic posture. *Vision* (Loewald, 1960) refers to the analyst's awareness that his patient's core is essentially organized toward the future and is striving towards greater organizational maturity. *Faith* (Bion, 1967) refers to the analyst's ability to sustain the belief that truth does exist and can be found. In that earlier essay, I highlighted the developmental antecedents and clinical application of these three attributes. I do not want to repeat that discourse here. What I want to do is to add how my originating from India (besides, of course, the specific formative experience of my childhood) adds a certain flavor to my analytic attitude.

Three features stand out. One is courage,[17] the other responsibility, and the third pertains to matters of money. The first two are related. By *courage*, I mean the capacity to assess the danger involved in a particular course of action and the mental willingness to bear certain risks since one considers that action to be right. Courage does not mean absence of fear. It means feeling fear and yet choosing to act according to one convictions. In my clinical work, I have found the accruing of courage over decades of experience. Some of it is simply due to ordinary age- and experience-based maturation. However, some of it emanates from the deeper assimilation of my Indian background into my clinical praxis. Take a look at the following clinical vignette, for instance.

Clinical Vignette 7

Judy Harris, a thin-skinned and shy, fearful but immensely needy young woman was in five-times-a-week analysis. From time to time, she felt a bit more confident of her acceptability to me. Usually this was a result of a piece of superego analysis, whereby the defensive nature of her inhibitions became more observable to her and whereby she learned of the childhood roots and current uses of terrifying inner injunctions. Mostly, she was afraid of overburdening me and immensely thankful for my attention. At other times, she expressed a need to see me more often, have longer sessions, meet me on her demand, and so on. Five times a week for 50 minutes certainly did not seem enough to her. I encouraged her to tell me more about all this. She revealed that as a child,

[17]I have discussed the nature of courage and its implications for psychoanalytic technique in my book, *Good Stuff* (2013).

she felt horribly rejected by her mother, who sternly discouraged any physical contact between them. She sobbed. We went on in this staccato fashion.

Then one day she revealed, fearfully and with some help from me that she has found out where I live and has driven by to take a look at my house. I experienced mixed feelings about this. Mostly, I felt fascination at this manner of transference deepening. The link between this behavior and her childhood wishes to touch her mother was clear to me. When I brought this to her attention, she too noticed the connection. However, the material did not deepen. Inquiries regarding what fantasies she had about my house, what or who did she really want to see, what did the house stand for, how looking at my house might have been a way of avoiding wishes to see me more fully (she was on the couch), yielded meagre results.

Gradually, the pattern of visiting my house became a regular one. Three, four times a week, including, at times, on weekends, she drove by the street on which I lived, slowing down as she passed my house, looking at it intently. Once in a while, from inside my house, I saw her driving by in her car. I felt a bit intruded upon but mostly, felt intrigued. I listened to the reports of these visits often but gained little further access to her inner world. I presented this situation to a study group, where some members expressed alarm and "not feeling frightened and angry". They suggested more active efforts at bringing this matter into the verbal discourse, getting at the underlying wishes of intruding upon the primal scene, cannibalism, whatever. One member recommended a prohibition of this behavior, thinking it will force the material back into the chamber of thought.

I found myself congenial to these ideas but not feeling truly alarmed; I was in no rush. A different approach presented itself to me. I was reminded that the patient wanted to see me more than five times a week and for longer sessions held at her demand. Was that a coercive control of me, behind which lurked the fear (wish) of having killed me during the intervals? Or, was it a developmental need? In other words, was the patient's wish to have more contact a hostile defense against deeper layers of even greater hostility, or was her going to my house an innovative way of having more sessions, without which she felt cognitively and emotionally disorganized? Two interventions were thus possible. One leaned toward interpreting the defensive and/or provocative nature of her actions. The other involved acknowledging the adaptive aspects of her behavior, which sought satisfaction of an ego need that I had failed to meet.

The issue is not which interventional direction is correct. The point I am trying to emphasize here is that I was courageous in bearing this situation partly because interpersonal closeness (even if it is a transference acting out) is more of an Indian character trait than a Western one. I found this patient's driving by my house not as disturbing as my colleagues did.

A related matter is that of *responsibility*. I feel that I am able and willing to assume an amount of responsibility for my patients that seems greater than my Western colleagues are comfortable with. Illustrations of it are difficult to give owing to confidentiality and medicolegal reasons but let us suppose a patient were to ask me to be the temporary custodian of a gun, cyanide poison, expensive jewelry, or a huge wad of cash, I might be willing to do so after an interpretative understanding of the situation reveals no better alternative. Also, I might respond to a late-night or weekend suicidal call by one of my patients *not* by referring him or her to an emergency room but by offering to see him or her myself. In a book of interviews by Hellinga et al. (2000), I answered their question about such a phone call from one of my patients in the following words:

> "I would stay on the phone for as long as it takes. If they are deadly serious, with a gun in their hand, threatening to blow their head off, I might ask them if they think it would be helpful for us to meet; that would simply be moving to another location, as it were, the kind of inconvenience that the patient is introducing anyway! There are times when such therapeutic actions are necessary. That offer in itself is so powerful and significant that it can rattle the patient and create a situation of hope, and diminish the anger, the revenge fantasies, etc. Secondly, if they are being obnoxious, I would ask them if they would object to giving me names or telephone numbers of relatives who I might call to help them. If they don't want to do that, then I would have to resort to other measures. I would say, "You know, by calling me, you have given me responsibility for what happens, so I am now going to call the police and make sure that they protect you and take you to the hospital". So it may be anything from calling the police to seeing them in person. If somebody is in bad trouble, there is no reason for not seeing them, even if it is at an odd hour of the day (or night). Other specialists like surgeons, internists, and gynecologists, do!" (p. 40).

Finally, there is the issue of money. My attitude about it is governed by an admixture of psychoanalytic principles and the Indian propensity to regard patients as *atithi* (the Sanskrit word for 'guest') and therefore extend all courtesy to them. To begin with, I do not charge three categories of individuals for the initial consultation (of one-two sessions): physicians, medical students, and Indians and their offspring.

I regard the first group as my siblings, the second as my children, and the third as my people.[18] Such existential kinship facilitates therapeutic alliance without altering the shape and context of future transferences, if I decide to take any one of these people in on-going treatment. My not charging Indians is essentially a reparative gesture of the remorse I feel over leaving India; I was not persecuted and left on my own will, thus, in effect, attacking the good internal object that my motherland was for me.

I also always carry a low-fee patient and almost never charge for missed sessions (unless there is grotesque exploitation and disregard of the frame by the patient). I am cognizant of Freud's (1913) firm stance on charging for missed sessions and of more recent 'explanations' (e.g., Ursano et al., 1998) of his position. However, in a radical departure from them, I have noted that:

> "To me, these explanations and the value system that underlies them appear harsh, self-serving, and devoid of physicianly kindness. I assert the following: (i) Freud's recommendations were developed nearly a 100 years ago when life's pace was slower, analyses were shorter, and authoritarian models of clinical work prevailed. These recommendations may have little applicability to the changed social and clinical milieu of today. (ii) Freud was a private practitioner with a large number of dependents and no other source of income beside clinical practice; his policy of charging for missed sessions reflected his personal situation and is less relevant to those practicing under different circumstances. (iii) While psychotherapy and psychoanalysis do require a certain asymmetry (with the patient revealing his inner world and the therapist withholding personal information), this asymmetry does not extend to all aspects of their work. Since the 'exigencies' of the therapist's life (e.g., illness, pregnancy, professional meetings) can and do impact upon the patient, it is morally unfair not to have the therapeutic frame accommodate the 'exigencies' of the patient's life. (iv) The assumption that the anger felt by the patient at being charged for a missed session is something that needs 'exploration' is also open to question. It blocks the consideration that the patient's anger at this situation might, at times, be legitimate" (2009c, p. 81).

Now, I acknowledge that my not charging for missed sessions is partly palatable because I have never been in private practice and have held a salaried, full-time job in a medical school. Variables of my personal history contribute to such a stance as well. However, I sense something Indian in it too. This might be traced to the internalization of the ancient Hindu tradition of treating an *atithi* (guest) with utmost humility as well as the incorporation

---

[18] Even the tendency to view others in terms of family is quintessentially Indian.

of the nineteenth and twentieth century customs of *Khush-ikhlaaqi* (good manners)[19] and *mehman-nawazi* (giving the best one has to the guest) of my birth city, Lucknow. Almost always, I give the benefit of doubt to the patient when it comes to money matters. I hasten to add that despite such financial lenience, I am no ascetic; I live well, enjoy traveling in business class, and have a reasonable collection of art and oriental carpets. My lack of financial anxiety is a reflection of the place my patients occupy in my heart, analytic or otherwise.

Technical Stance

While most individuals who seek clinical help from me do so because of being referred by therapists whom they respect or because they have heard me speak at some conference or have ready something I have published, there is a small group of patients in my practice—say, about 20%—whose choice of me as an analyst emanates from a deep and unmourned attachment to a Chinese housekeeper or an African American nanny. A partial 'reunion' with the lost object—or, to put it in Leo Stone's (1960) terms 'resemblance'—seems necessary for them to work through the complex feelings attached to the early caretaker who often had abruptly and prematurely left them (see also Coles, 1915, in this regard).

Given this, I generally maintain a 'low-keyed' curiosity about my patients' choice of me as their analyst. Asking direct questions in this regard is hardly ever helpful. It can drive the significant material, if it does exist, away from consciousness and behind socially appropriate ego defenses. Also, this gentle skepticism regarding the patient's choice should be tempered by the recognition that, at times, such choices have no 'deep' significance at all. At other times, a seemingly mundane, early reference to ethnic matters might be the first hint of major transferences lying in wait.

Clinical Vignette 8

Dr Robert Purple, a 40-year-old internist, sought consultation with me for some phobic anxieties. He came from a suburb and was unfamiliar with downtown Philadelphia. In his first session with me, he said that he was not favorably impressed by the town, and added with a snicker that "too many Vietnamese and Cambodian vendors seem to have moved in here." When I noted the potential allusion in this remark to me, the patient quickly denied any ethnic anxieties regarding our working together.

---

[19] I have elsewhere (Akhtar, 2011a) written about the role of good manners in psychoanalytic technique.

Once the patient was well-settled in analysis, however, he began to display considerable prejudice against Asians. He regarded Indians as being especially incompetent. Still later, he sheepishly revealed that he had deliberately sought an analyst who would be incompetent so that he would not be hurt too much in undergoing analysis. In other words, my expected incompetence so that he would save him from coming to terms with his shame-laden aspects. Projection of his own feelings of being weak and incompetent vis-à-vis his older brother and father were gradually discerned, as were hidden masochistic desires to be mistreated.

While in the beginning a patiently curious attitude is ideal, the demands made by some patients call for limit setting from the outset. Only then can an investigative collaboration be set in motion.

Clinical Vignette 9

Rebecca Cohen, a young Jewish internist, whose father was a Holocaust survivor, called me, seeking psychoanalysis. She was well-informed about analysis and had been given my name by an elderly Jewish analyst. While setting an appointment on the phone, she asked me: "Are you an Arab?" I responded by saying that while I was interested in her questions and what lay behind it, I could not answer it on a factual basis. I added that if we were going to undertake any kind of in-depth work together, my real life situation was less important than what she made of it in her mind. The patient, however, persisted, saying "look, I am a devout Jew and an ardent Zionist. I know that if you are an Arab, your sympathies in the Israeli-Palestinian conflict will lie with the Palestinians. And I am not about to give my money to someone who will support terrorism against my own people." I was taken aback by the sadomasochistic proclivity under a thin patina of ethnic rationalization. I responded by repeating what I had said and adding that if she found herself will to tolerate ambiguity and investigate what had already begun to take place, then perhaps we could meet. Otherwise, she might have to go elsewhere. She came for her appointment and did enter analysis with me.

In the subsequent 6 years or so, the patient, who turned out to be neither a devout Jew nor an ardent Zionist, underwent a rather stormy analysis.[20] Provocative limit-testing and recall through enactment pervaded the early phase. Three themes took center stage, in succession though criss-crossing each other: (1) The Holocaust and her

[20] In fact, it was towards the end of her analysis that she began to be comfortable with her ethnic identity. For the first time, after years, she went to a synagogue and, during the services, found herself thanking me in her heart!

contradictory identifications with her father's survivor guilt (Niederland, 1968) and his persecutor's sadism, (2) the separation guilt (Modell, 1984) involving a depressed mother, and (3) a negative oedipal defense against guilt-ridden positive oedipal strivings. These shifts, interestingly, were associated with changing perceptions of my ethnicity: first, an Arab (equated in her mind with a Nazi), then an Indian Muslim (equated in her mind with a Jew since both represented minorities), and finally, a reasonably assimilated immigrant North-American.

These two vignettes illustrate the admixture of defensive and fantasy-based motivations for seeking a culturally different, immigrant analyst. Shifting transferences, such as those described above, and their corresponding ethnic metaphors warrant that the analyst constantly scan the associative material for disguised and displaced references to his ethnicity or race (Abbasi, 1997; Holmes, 1992; Leary, 1995). If the analyst comes from a country or region known to be culturally quite different and especially if he has a skin color that is different from the patient, then he is certainly "more than just a blank screen, and his. . .color will pull forth a rich variety of projections and stereotypes" (Tang and Gardener, 1999, p. 8; see also Ticho, 1971). Holmes (1992) notes that such "points of access to a patient's transferences" (p. 8) give rise to rich associations that need to be carefully deciphered. However, this activity should not occur at the cost of sacrificing interest in other meanings of the patient's material.

One other point. The analyst's ethnicity not only mobilizes transferences, it can be used by the patient in the service of resistance as well. The homoethnic patient might use it for nostalgic collusion that seeks to preclude deeper investigation of certain themes, usually of an aggressive nature (Akhtar, 2011–Immigration). The heteroethnic patient might use the analyst's ethnicity as a rationalization for accepting or not accepting his interpretations.

Clinical Vignette 10

Jack Lieberman, a deeply traumatized but highly successful businessman in his mid-sixties, suffered from chronic self-loathing and from uncertainty despite frequent accolades from esteemed others and almost daily hob-nobbing with renowned members of society. He had grown up with constant ridicule and abuse by his somewhat sociopathic older brother who, in Jack's perception, was secretly admired by his parents. Moreover, Jack never felt truly appreciated by his parents, no matter what he achieved or accomplished. As an adult, he often derided himself as being inferior to others, unable to love, have empathy for this or that person, and forgive others for their blemishes. He dismissed his own cognitive and linguistic talents, especially in the realm of administration and business negotiations, with an air of nonchalance, if not derision.

He experienced disbelief when his wife praised his appearance and called him a 'good man.'

In the same vein, when I made any intervention that portrayed him in a positive light, he quickly dismissed it by attributing it to my 'Indian goodness.' Behind such inability to accept the interpretation lurked enormous hunger for love as well as guilt over the grasping and hostile edge to that hunger.

A few words about countertransference also seem warranted. There is something special about my work with *Indian patients* because such patients are few and far between in my clinical practice and often have cultural similarities with me. This has both positive and negative aspects. On the positive side, bringing up a mythological figure or referring to a Bollywood movie or reciting a snippet of an Urdu poem deepens the working alliance with them. On the negative side, the risk of 'nostalgic collusion' (Akhtar, 2011b) and displacement of aggression to outside—mostly American figures ('them')—can detract from deep analytic work. *With immigrant patients from nations other than India,* (e.g., Greece, Italy, and Russia), the intuitive knowledge of the trauma of dislocation provides the cement for our bonding, though not without the above-mentioned risks. With *patients who are United States-born citizens,* both the polarities of built-in empathy and undue indulgence appear less intense and the analytic process stays on a more even keel. My Indian self does not go to sleep, though. Occasionally, a song from a Bollywood movie, seen long ago, pops up in my mind and catalyzes self-analysis which, in turn, enriches my work with the patient.

Clinical Vignette 11

Alice McGuire, a very attractive woman, was once talking about her desire to make love with me and especially to be naked in front of me and have me admire her body. Alice had lost her mother at the peak of the oedipal phase and had experienced her stepmother (who came on the scene some 2 years later) as cold and devoid of sensuality.

As Alice expressed this desire, an old Hindi movie song (*Juhi Ki Kali, meri laadli; naazoN Ki pali, meri laadli*) popped up in my mind. In the movie, Dil Ek Mandir (1963), which I saw some 40 years ago, the song is sung by an adoring mother to her 4-year-old daughter. Becoming aware of this, I quietly wondered if I were defending against an erotic countertransference by thinking of a mother-child rather than a man-woman interaction. Another possibility was that the longing for mother's admiration undergirded Alice's desire that I admire her naked body. Questioning myself along these lines led to deeper self-contact and furthered my capacity to work with my patient.

Fascinatingly, a few days later, Alice brought up the fantasy of dressing up in a gorgeous outfit to attract me. Just as she expressed this desire, I found myself humming (inaudibly, of course) a song from the 1965 Bollywood movie, *Mere Sanam*. This song – *Humdum mere, maan bhi jaao, kehna mere pyar ka* – (literally translated: O beloved one, listen to the longings of my heart) was sung in the movie by a desperately smitten hero for a beautiful woman that he had fallen in love with. Clearly, I was resonating with Alice's erotic feelings towards me. What later occurred to me was that her fantasy of taking her clothes off in front of me did not mobilize erotic feelings in me but her fantasy of putting on beautiful clothes did. A question then arose in my mind: did this difference reflect something unanalyzed within me or was it the result of a proper attunement to the patient's psyche at that moment? Or, was there something typically Indian in my being 'turned on' only (or mainly) by the aim-inhibited expression of her sensuality?

To summarize then, in this section of the paper, I have discussed how my Indian self gets involved and entangled in creating the office space, the language, the therapeutic attitude, and the technical posture for my conducting psychoanalysis. Time to conclude, now.

CONCLUSION

In this contribution, I have surveyed how India, as an internalized good object and as an organizing idiom of discourse, has enriched my analytic career. Although wide-ranging, the essay has omitted three areas of overlap between India and psychoanalysis in my life. These include:

- My experience as an Indian undergoing analysis with North American Jewish analysts who did not know my mother-tongue and had never been to India.
- My publications pertaining to India. Among these, the most prominent ones are the edited volume, *Freud Along the Ganges* (Akhtar, 2005), which contains multifaceted essays on the people and culture of India, and the solo-authored, *The Book of Emotions* (Akhtar, 2012), which explicates twenty-six human emotions with the help of Hindu mythology, India's history, Urdu poetry, and scenes from Bollywood movies.
- My educational efforts, especially my co-founding (with Dr Jennifer Bonovitz) of the South Asian American Forum at the Psychoanalytic Center of Philadelphia (1996), helping organize the Center for Psychoanalytic Studies at Delhi University (2005), twice-a-year teaching workshops for a group of psychoanalytic therapists in New Delhi, especially those associated with Ambedkar University (2010 – present), and sponsoring the publication of papers by many Indian psychoanalysts in Western journals and IPA-sponsored edited books.

To have addressed these areas in detail would have taken far more space than this paper allows; it may warrant a separate paper in the future. I have therefore restricted my focus to matters of theory (especially those pertaining to the death instinct and the psychoanalytic discomfort with religion) and clinical practice (especially the realms of the clinical space, analyst's mother-tongue, therapeutic attitude, and some aspects of technique). My hope in doing so is to inform my American colleagues and psychoanalytic progeny of my veracity, to offer my non-Indian immigrant colleagues and progeny a parallel world of camaraderie, and to inspire my Indian psychoanalytic colleagues and progeny towards a more authentic 'going-on-being' (Winnicott, 1956) as psychoanalysts. To what extent I have succeeded in achieving these goals, only the readers of this contribution can decide. I can only put my feelings at this concluding juncture in the form of a couplet I wrote a few months ago:

"Jo baat such hai, Kabhi to bataayi jaayegi.
Meri kahani bhi us din sunaaye jaayegi"

Literally, "The truth shall one day be revealed, for sure. And it is then that my story will also be told to everyone". I am glad that the day I was waiting for has arrived. Well, more or less!

FURTHER READING

1. Abbasi A. Whose side are you on? Muslim psychoanalysts treating non-Muslim patients. In: S Akhtar (Ed). The Crescent and the Couch: Cross-currents between Islam and Psychoanalysis. New York: Other Press; 2008. pp. 335-50.
2. Akhtar S. Immigration and Identity: Turmoil, Treatment, and Transformation. Northvale, NJ: Jason Aronson; 1999.
3. Akhtar S. From mental pain through manic defense to mourning. In: S Akhtar (Ed). Three Faces of Mourning: Melancholia, Manic defense, and moving on. Northvale, NJ: Jason Aronson; 2001. pp. 95-115.
4. Akhtar S. Freud along the Ganges: Psychoanalytic Reflections on the People and Culture of India. New York: Other Press; 2005.
5. Akhtar S. Four roadblocks in approaching Masud Khan. Psychoanal Q. 2007; 76:991-5.
6. Akhtar S (2009a). Comprehensive dictionary of psychoanalysis. London, UK: Karnac.
7. Akhtar S (2009b). The damaged core: Origins, dynamics, manifestations, and treatment. Lanham Md.: Jason Aronson.
8. Akhtar S (2009c). Turning points in dynamic psychotherapy: Initial assessment, boundaries, money, disruptions, and suicidal crises. London, UK: Karnac.
9. Akhtar S (2011a). Matters of life and death: Psychoanalytic reflections. London, UK: Karnac.
10. Akhtar S (2011b). Immigration and acculturation: Mourning, adaptation, and the next generation. Lanham, Md.: Jason Aronson.

11. Akhtar S (2012a). The Book of Emotions. New Delhi, India: Lotus Collection.
12. Akhtar S (2012b). Good stuff: Generosity, resilience, humility, gratitude, forgiveness, and sacrifice. Lanham, Md.: Jason Aronson.
13. Akhtar S. Psychoanalytic listening: Methods, limits, and innovations. London, UK: Karnac; 2013.
14. Akhtar S, Parens H (Eds). Does God help? Developmental and clinical aspects of religious belief. Lanham, Md.: Jason Aronson; 2001.
15. Bach S. On narcissistic state of consciousness. Internat. J. Psychoanal. 1997;58:209-33.
16. Bion W (1962). Learning from experience. London, UK: Karnac; 1984.
17. Bion W. (1965). Transformations. London, UK: Karnac; 1984.
18. Bion W. Notes on memory and desire. Psychoanal. Forum. 1967;2:272-3.
19. Bion W (1970). Attention and interpretation. London, UK: Karnac, 1984.
20. Bolognini S (2008). Secret passages: The theory and technique of interpsychic relations (trans. G. Atkinson). New York: Routledge; 2011.
21. Carpelan H. On the importance of the setting in the psychoanalytic situation. Scand. Psychoanal Rev. 1981;4:151-61.
22. Chasseguet-Smirgel J. Creativity and perversion. New York: Norton; 1984.
23. Coles P. The shadow of the second mother: Nurses and nannies in theories of infant development. London, UK: Routledge; 2015.
24. Coltart N. Slouching towards Bethlehem and further psychoanalytic explorations. London, UK: Free Association Books; 1986.
25. Cooper J. Speak of me as I am: The life and work of Masud Khan. London, UK: Karnac; 1993.
26. Eigen M. The area of faith in Winnicott, Lacan, and Bion. Internat J Psychoanal. 1981;62:413-33.
27. Eissler K. Death drive, ambivalence, and narcissism. Psychoanal. Study of the Child. 1971;26:25-78.
28. Faiz FA. Dast-e-Saba. Lahore, Pakistan: Urdu Adab; 1952.
29. Fayek A. From interpretation to the death instinct. Internat. Rev. Psycho-Anal. 1980;7:447-57.
30. Feldman M. Some views on the manifestation of the death instinct in clinical work. Internat J Psycho-Anal. 2000;81:53-65.
31. Feldman M. Manifestations on the death instinct in the consulting room. In: B Joseph (Ed). Doubt, conviction and the analytic process: Selected papers of Michael Feldman. London, UK: Routledge; 2009. pp. 96-117.
32. Ferenczi S (1911). On obscene words. In: Contributions to psycho-analysis. (trans. E. Jones). Boston, Mass.: Richard G. Budger; 1916. pp. 112-30.
33. Freud S. On beginning the treatment. In J. Strachey, ed. and trans., The standard edition of the complete psychological works of Sigmund Freud, 24 vols. London: Hogarth Press, 1953-1974. 1913;12:123-144.
34. Freud, S. (1915-1916). Introductory lectures on psychoanalysis. Parts I and II. Standard ed. 15, 16.
35. Freud S. From the history of an infantile neurosis. Standard ed. 1918;17:1-122.
36. Freud S. Beyond the pleasure principle. Standard ed.1920;18:7-64.
37. Freud S. The ego and the id. Standard ed.1923;19:1-66.
38. Freud S. The economic problem of masochism. Standard ed.1924;19:155-70.

39. Freud S. Inhibitions, symptoms, and anxiety. Standard ed. 1926;20:77-175.
40. Freud S. The future of an illusion. Standard ed.1927;21:5-56.
41. Freud S. Civilization and its discontents. Standard ed. 1930;21:64-145.
42. Freud S. Analysis terminable and interminable. Standard ed.1937;23:209-255.
43. Freud S [1938]. An outline of psychoanalysis. Standard ed. 1940;23:139-207.
44. Gay P. Freud: A life for our time. New York: Norton; 1988.
45. Ghalib AUK (1841). Diwan-e-Ghalib. New Delhi, India: Maktaba Jamia; 1972.
46. Goldman S. Sigmund Freud's Briefe an seine patientin Anna W. Vest. Jahrbuch Psychoanal.1985;17:293-294.
47. Green A. The death drive, negative narcissism and the disobjectalising function. In: The work of the negative (trans. A. Weller). London, UK: Free Association Books; 1999.
48. Hellinga G, Van Luyn B, Dalewijk HJ. Personalities: Master clinicians confront the treatment of borderline personality disorder. Amsterdam, The Netherlands: Boom Publishers; 2000.
49. Hoffman MT. Toward mutual recognition: Relational psychoanalysis and the Christian narrative. London, UK: Routledge; 2011.
50. Holmes DE. Race and transference in psychoanalysis and psychotherapy. Internat J Psychoanal. 1992;73:1-11.
51. Jacobson E. The self and the object world. New York: International Universities Press; 1964.
52. Jones E. The life and work of Sigmund Freud, Vol. III. New York: Basic Books; 1957
53. Kakar S. Re-reading Freud on religion in Hindu, India. In: MK. O'Neil, S Akhtar (Eds). On Freud's "The future of an illusion". London, UK: Karnac; 2007. pp. 224-36.
54. Kernberg O. The concept of the death drive: A clinical perspective. Internat J Psychoanal. 2009;90:1009-23.
55. Kersun J, Silberman E. The psychiatric office. In: JA Lazarus (Ed). Entering private practice. Washington DC: American Psychiatric Publishing; 2005. pp. 37-54.
56. Khan M. The concept of cumulative trauma. Psychoanal Study of the Child. 1963;18:286-306.
57. Khan M (1969). On symbiotic omnipotence. In: The privacy of the self. New York: International Universities Press; 1974. pp. 82-92.
58. Khan M. On lying fallow. In: Hidden selves: Between theory and practice in psychoanalysis. New York: International Universities Press; 1983. pp. 183-88.
59. Klein M (1933). The early development of conscience in the child. In Love, guilt, and reparation, and other works, 1921-1945. New York: Free Press; 1984. pp. 262-89.
60. Klein M (1935). A contribution to the psychogenesis of manic depressive states. In: Love, guilt, and reparation, and other works, 1921-1945. New York: Free Press; 1975. pp. 262-89.
61. Klein, M. (1952). Some theoretical conclusions regarding the emotional life of the infant. In Envy and gratitude, and other works, 1946-1963. New York: Free Press; 1975. pp. 61-93.
62. Kaplan L. Oneness and separateness: From infant to individual. New York: Simon and Schuster; 1977.

63. Killingmo B. Conflict and deficit: Implications for technique. Internat J Psycho-Anal. 1989;70:65-79.
64. Leary K (1995). Interpreting in the dark: Race and ethnicity in psychoanalytic psychotherapy. Psychoanal Psychol. 1989;12:127-40.
65. Lewin B. The psychoanalysis of elation. New York: Norton; 1950.
66. Lichtenstein H. The dilemma of human identity: Notes on self-transformation, self-objectivation, and metamorphosis. J Amer Psychoanal Assoc.1963; 11:173-223.
67. Loewald H. On the therapeutic action of psychoanalysis. J Amer Psychoanal Assoc. 1960;41:16-33.
68. López-Corvo RE. The dictionary of the work of WR Bion. London, UK: Karnac Books; 2005.
69. Mahler M. A study of the separation and individuation process and its possible application to borderline phenomena in the psychoanalytic situation. Psychoanal Study of the Child. 1971;26:403-24.
70. Mahler M, Bergman A, Pine F. The psychological birth of the human infant. New York: Basic Books; 1975.
71. Masson JM (Ed). The complete letters of Sigmund Freud to Wilhelm Fliess. Cambridge, Mass.: Harvard University Press; 1985.
72. Modell AH. On having the right to a life: An aspect of the superego's development. Internat J Psychoanal. 1965;46:323-31.
73. Neri C. What is the function of faith and trust in psychoanalysis? Internat J Psychoanal. 2005;86:79-97.
74. Nicholi AM Jr. The question of God: CS Louis and Sigmund Freud debate God, love, sex, and the meaning of life. New York: Free Press; 2002.
75. Niederland WG. Clinical observations on the "survivor syndrome." Internat J Psychoanal. 1968;49:313-5.
76. O'Neil, MK, Akhtar S (Eds). On Freud's "The Future of an Illusion." London, UK: Karnac; 2008.
77. Paterson M. Obituary: Masud Khan. Free Associations. 1991;21:109-11.
78. Pine F. Diversity and direction in psychoanalytic technique. New Haven, Conn.: Yale University Press; 1997.
79. Rao D. Manifestations of God in India: A transference pantheon. In: S Akhtar (Ed). Freud along the Ganges: Psychoanalytic reflections on the people and culture of India. New York: Other Press; 2005. pp. 271-308.
80. Roland A. In: search of self in India and Japan: Toward a cross-cultural psychology. Princeton NJ.: Princeton University Press; 1988.
81. Rosenfeld H. A clinical approach to the psychoanalytic theory of the life and death instincts: An investigation into aggressive aspects of narcissism. Internat J Psycho-anal. 1971;52:169-78.
82. Russell R. The famous Ghalib. New Delhi, India. Roli; 2000.
83. Schmidt-Hellerau C. Surviving in absence: On the preservative and death drives and their clinical utility. Psychoanal Q. 2000;75:1057-95.
84. Sen A. The argumentative Indian: Writings on Indian history, culture, and identity. London, UK: Penguin; 2005.
85. Settlage CF. Defenses evoked by early childhood loss: Their impact on life-span development. In: S Akhtar (Ed). Three faces of mourning: Melancholia, manic defense, and moving on. Northvale, NJ.: Jason Aronson; 2001. pp. 47-93.

86. Shafii M. Sufi perspective on human suffering and its relief. In: S Akhtar (Ed). The crescent and the couch: Cross-currents between Islam and psychoanalysis Lanham, Md.: Jason Aronson; 2018. pp. 161-80.
87. Shengold L. A variety of narcissistic pathology stemming from parental weakness. Psychoanal Q. 1991;60:86-92.
88. Stone L. The psychoanalytic situation. New York: International Universities Press; 1960.
89. Stone L Reflections on the psychoanalytic concept of aggression. Psychoanal Q. 1971;40:195-244.
90. Tang NM, Gardner J. Race, culture, and psychotherapy: Transference to minority therapists. Psychoanal Q. 1999;68:1-20.
91. Ticho G. Cultural aspects of transference and countertransference. Bull Menninger Clinic. 1971;35:313-26.
92. Ursano RJ, Sonnenberg SM, Lazar SG. Concise guide to psychodynamic psychotherapy. Washington DC: American Psychiatric Press; 1998.
93. Vallabheneni MR. Advaita Vedanta, psychoanalysis and the self. In: S Akhtar (Ed). Freud along the Ganges: Psychoanalytic reflections on the people and culture of India. New York: Other Press; 2005. pp. 359-93.
94. Winnicott DW. Transitional objects and transitional phenomena. Internat J Psycho-Anal. 1953;34:89-97.
95. Winnicott DW (1956). Primary maternal preoccupation. In: Collected papers: Through paediatrics to psychoanalysis. New York: Basic Books, 1958. pp. 300-5.
96. Winnicott DW. The theory of parent-infant relationship. Internat J Psychoanal. 1960;41:585-95.
97. Winnicott DW (1962). Ego integration in child development. In: Maturational processes and the facilitating environment. New York: International Universities Press; 1965. pp. 45-53.
98. Winnicott DW (1968). Use of an object and relating through identifications. In: Playing and reality. London, UK: Tavistock, 1971. pp. 86-94.

Epilogue

11 CHAPTER

Future Directions and Recommendations

Geetha Desai, Pratap Sharan, Vinay Kumar, Salman Akhtar

Psychotherapy is an essential component of the treatment of various mental health problems and is also crucial for persons who are seeking to improve their mental wellbeing. In a transitional society like ours, the need for psychotherapy is immense. We have been following various schools of psychotherapy in varied formats, and the growth of psychotherapy in India has fluctuated with time.

The practice of psychotherapy by psychiatrists is often limited to various teaching and training institutes. Still, there has been a changing trend with private practitioners considering the importance of the same. There could be multiple reasons for this: The number of psychiatrists practicing psychotherapy needs to be in keeping with the demands for psychotherapy. There is an ongoing debate on who should be doing psychotherapy and whether psychiatrists are qualified enough to do psychotherapy. The biggest challenge has been the fidelity of the psychotherapy practice, and there needs to be more clarity between counseling and psychotherapy. Despite evidence on the biological basis for psychotherapy, many psychiatrists do not consider this as an essential area. Psychotherapeutic psychiatry (a word used by Dr Pratap Sharan) might be a stepping stone for psychotherapy practice.

Training in psychotherapy is highly varied during the residency/postgraduate training program, with only a few institutions and medical colleges in India following a comprehensive psychotherapy program. There is a need to emphasize the need for training in psychotherapy for all postgraduate students and become an integral part of their MD program. This can be achieved only by involving the agencies which regulate the course training.

Most psychotherapies currently being followed have originated in the West, and the evidence for the same has also been conducted predominantly in the West. As elucidated in the book, we need to use the cultural contexts and develop and test the models of psychotherapy in the Indian context. Research evidence for psychotherapies in India needs to be considered a prominent research area. The Indian Psychiatric Society can consider this an essential piece of research and emphasize on the policymakers to fund research focusing on this area.

Three important caveats must, however, be entered:

1. First, those spearheading efforts to strengthen psychotherapy should resist a surgical East-West separation in conceptualization and praxis. Geocultural differences exist and need to be investigated, understood, and assimilated in the corpus of theory and technique. But it should be remembered that such divergences mostly involve child-rearing norms, hence modal relational patterns and character styles. They do not affect 'metapsychology' or the understanding of how the mind functions (e.g., the conscious-unconscious compartmentalization, intrapsychic conflict, defense mechanisms); these discoveries, even though originally made in the West, are universally applicable and need retention in models that are being or might in future be, evolved in the East. A close study of how this has been attempted in Eastern nations other than India (especially China, Japan, and South Korea) might provide much food for thought here.
2. The second caveat pertains to the development of a more or less uniform didactic curriculum in psychotherapy for psychiatry residents in India. The first step in this process is to solicit and pool the curricula that already exist and update them in light of contemporary developments in the field. Here, the advisory input of Indian-born psychotherapists and psychoanalysts from the UK, USA, Canada, and Australia can be immensely beneficial. Possessing cultural sensitivity as well as up-to-date knowledge of the modern psychotherapy literature [be it Cognitive Behavior Therapy (CBT); Dialectical Behavior Therapy (DBT); Transference Focused Therapy (TFP), or psychoanalysis], these colleagues should be invited to serve as consultants on a Psychotherapy Curriculum Development Committee established by the Indian Psychiatric Society. Following the evolution and acceptance of the document prepared by this group on which practitioners in India should, of course, also serve, a pilot study of its actual execution (in the form of didactic and clinical teaching) should be undertaken. Yet another step might be psychotherapy workshops, based upon portions of this curriculum, to be held on a quarterly basis for regional psychiatric trainees. Invited teachers of Indian origin from abroad should lead or co-lead such workshops with the aim not only of imparting pertinent knowledge but also cultivating aspiring teachers among the rising group within India. Needless to say the feasibility of accomplishing such goals via modern electronic media of communication should also be explored and deployed.
3. Finally, attempts to enhance and enrich psychotherapy training and practice in India must be fearless and unshackle themselves from the bounds of psychiatry; dialogue must be started with nonmedical psychotherapists and psychoanalysts to see what common mental health conceptualizing and delivery models are waiting there to be evolved.

From a public health perspective, to make psychotherapy accessible to large sections of the population, there is a need for training at 4 levels: (1) Training of master trainers, (2) training of psychotherapists, (3) training in psychotherapy for all mental health professionals, and (4) training in psychotherapy for select sets of community health workers. Currently, psychotherapy training is available at level 2 (becoming a psychotherapist) from the Indian Psychoanalytical Society and National Institute of Mental Health and NeuroSciences (NIMHANS) (1-year full-time clinical fellowship in CBT for postgraduates who have completed their MPhil in Clinical Psychology from an Rehabilitation Council of India (RCI) recognized institute) and level 3 for clinical psychologists, psychiatrists, and other mental health professionals at a few institutions. Sensitization workshops are offered by the Indian Psychiatric Society and the Indian Association for CBT.

The main barrier on the supply side is inadequate resources at the first two levels and lack of time at the latter two levels. On the demand side, economic, literacy, and cultural issues may need to be addressed. However, considering the huge supply crunch, the demand side barriers may be less salient, but they distort supply towards the affluent Westernized subpopulations rather than provision based on need.

There is a need to scale up training at all 4 levels as each level becomes a resource for the next. In particular, there is a need to develop/adapt packages that can be delivered through task sharing/stepped care approaches. Another approach to making psychotherapy accessible is to develop self-help materials drawn from evidence-based psychological treatment principles (self-help books or audiovisual materials; online or app-based self-help interventions).

It is time to pay attention to psychotherapy training, research and practice in India and the impetus for this need to form organizations, practitioners and societies in Psychiatry.

Index